# RENAL PROBLEMS

## A Critical Care Nursing Focus

Mary Jackle, R.N., M.S.
*Director, Critical Care Project*

Claire Rasmussen, R.N.
*Renal Nurse Specialist*

Metropolitan Medical Center
*Minneapolis, Minnesota*

***Renal Problems: A Critical Care Nursing Focus***



Library of Congress Cataloging in Publication Data

Jackle, Mary
Renal problems.

1. Kidneys—Diseases—Nursing. 2. Kidneys—Diseases—Case studies. I. Rasmussen, Claire, joint author. II. Title. [DNLM: 1. Critical care—Nursing. 2. Kidney diseases—Nursing. WY164 J124r] RC902.J32 1980 616.6'1 79-9498

ISBN 0-87619-408-0

Prentice-Hall International, Inc., London
Prentice-Hall of Australia, Pty., Ltd. Sydney
Prentice-Hall of India Private Limited, New Delhi
Prentice-Hall of Japan, Inc., Tokyo
Prentice-Hall of Southeast Asia Pte. Ltd., Singapore
Whitehall Books, Limited, Petone, New Zealand

Printed in the United States of America

80 81 82 83 84 85 86 10 9 8 7 6 5 4 3 2 1

# CONTENTS

To my parents, Marian and John Jackle
M.J.

To Mary
and
To Richard and Scott
C.R.

# Preface

The content of this book evolved during three years of teaching registered nurses and senior nursing students in basic Critical Care Nursing courses. Our aim is to assist readers in making appropriate nursing decisions in the care of acutely ill patients with renal problems. Such nursing decisions rely on a broad understanding of renal function and the results of pathological processes.

The text is organized to accomplish the following goals:

Section 1 Review anatomy of the kidney, and the causes of renal disease.

Section 2 Explain the key concepts of physiology and pathology underlying renal disease processes, and describe parameters of a systematic nursing assessment of renal function.

Section 3 Use representative case studies of acutely ill patients to demonstrate the clinical course, frequently occurring nursing needs, appropriate nursing goals and intervention for renal problems. Purposes and principles of dialysis and transplantation are discussed, as well as implications for nursing care of the patient.

The reader will need additional study, instruction and practice to learn about the wide range of renal diseases; the implications of chronic renal problems; the ethical, legal and social issues involved; and specific nursing routines and procedures in local use.

This book is intended for registered nurses who are studying critical care nursing in a basic course or independently, nurse-orientees in critical care units, and upper-division level nursing students. We assume readers have knowledge of the basics of anatomy and physiology of each body system, pharmacology, medical and surgical nursing and nursing processes, and that it is at the level we have observed in a majority of our students.

The programmed instruction method was chosen to reflect our classroom experience with active, inquisitive learners, because it stimulates the reader to reason, participate and evaluate progress. Each chapter begins with learner objectives and an outline of content. A brief summary follows each major part of the chapter, to encourage the reader's synthesis of information.

We would like to thank

Our teachers for sharing their knowledge and encouraging us to create

Our students for testing the program and helping us to grow as instructors

Our patients for teaching us about resourcefulness and courage

Our colleagues at Metropolitan Medical Center and the Regional Kidney Disease Program for their assistance and advice, especially: Mary E.

Jones, R.N., M.S., Director of Nursing, for providing the time resources, personal encouragement and administrative support for this project; Carol Wicklund for competently typing the manuscript through all its revisions; and Marney Halligan, Jean Field and Marilyn Bergstrom for graciously taking on extra work to give us time to write, and for their friendship.

Mary Jackle
Claire Rasmussen

# Introduction

You are about to begin studying a programmed text. This kind of instruction may be new to you, so please read the following instructions.

The book is designed so that each chapter builds on the previous one, so start at the beginning of the book, at Frame 1. Skipping around in the book would be confusing.

Each frame must be studied carefully because it represents one step in a series of concepts. Material is divided into small portions of information, and explanations have been pared down, so that the frames may be quickly understood. As you work on the book, cover the answer column with a strip of paper. Each frame will first give you information and then ask you questions about that information. You should check your answer with the one given. If you gave a wrong answer, you may have scanned the frame too quickly and missed details or subtle points. Return to the frame and study it again to see where your error occurred. You will also find information presented in *panels.* The panels provide illustrations and a more detailed explanation of certain points. At the end of each major section of the chapter, a summary frame will help you review your learning.

Once you have gotten used to this method, you will be able to progress at a pace that is appropriate for you. Tests have indicated that our students learned the content well with an average of 15–20 hours of study. Now it is your turn!

Executive Producer: Richard A. Weimer
Production Editor: Marlise Reidenbach
Illustrations: Don Sellers, Wayne R. Lewis
Cover and Text Design: Laura Lammens

# Section I
# Review

# CHAPTER 1

# ANATOMY REVIEW

## Introduction

Before studying renal problems, it would be helpful to review the anatomy of the urinary system. After completing this chapter you will be confident that you can

1. Recognize the components of the urinary system
2. Identify selected microscopic structures of the kidney
3. Name the components of the nephron
4. List the two kidney functions that are vital to life.

## Frame 1

Identify the structures labeled A through E on this figure:

A. ______________

B. ______________

C. ______________

D. ______________

E. ______________

A. Adrenal gland

B. Kidney

C. Ureter

D. Bladder

E. Urethra

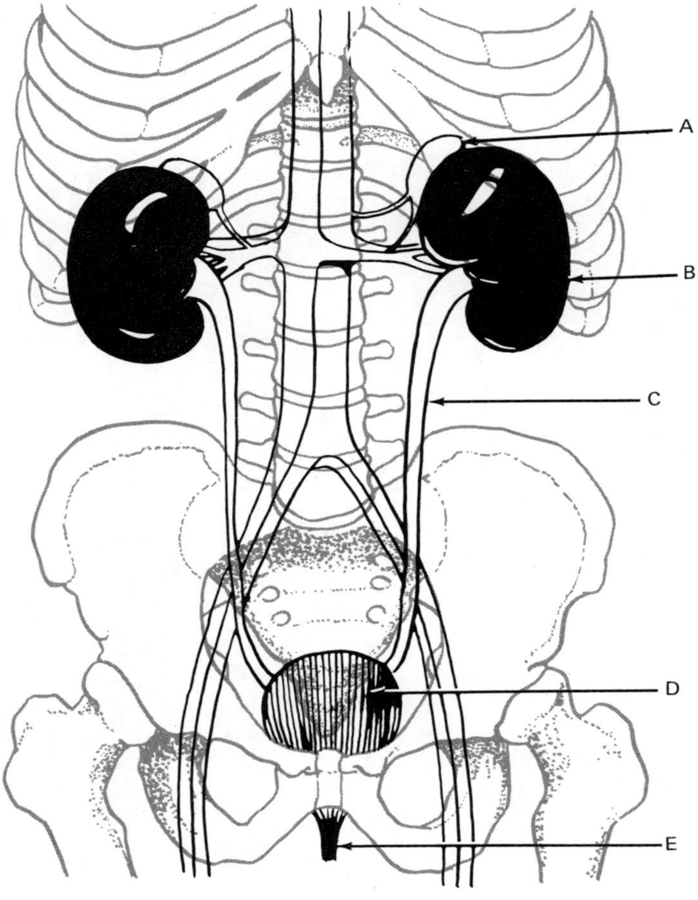


Figure 1

If you had any answers wrong, see Frame 4.

## Frame 2

Identify the structures labeled A through H on the longitudinal section of a kidney shown in this figure:

A. ______________

B. ______________

C. ______________

D. ______________

E. ______________

F. ______________

G. ______________

H. ______________

A. Renal pelvis

B. Cortex

C. Medulla

D. Calyx

E. Apex of pyramid (papilla)

F. Pyramid

G. Ureter

H. Renal artery and vein

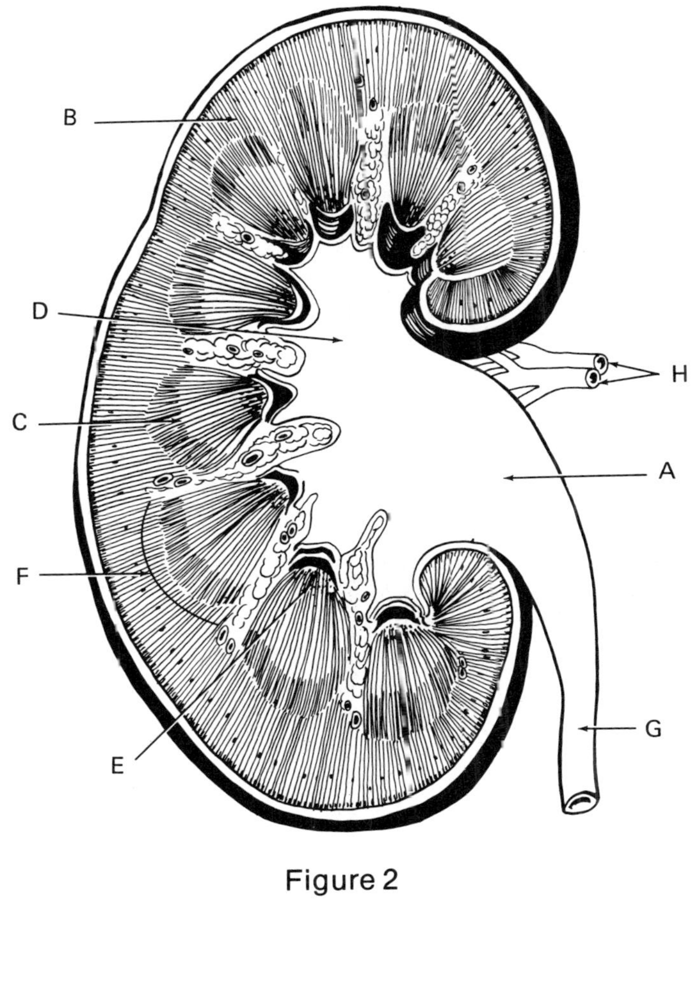


Figure 2

Fill in the blanks with the correct words to complete these statements:

1. An ____________ gland is located on the upper aspect of each kidney.
2. The renal artery, vein, lymphatic vessels and nerves enter and leave the kidney through the ____________.
3. In longitudinal section, two distinct areas are observed in the kidney: an inner area called the ____________ and an outer area called the ____________.

1. adrenal
2. hilus
3. medulla
   cortex

If you have questions about these structures, see Frames 5, 6 and 7.

## Frame 3

Identify the structures labeled A through D on the nephron shown in figure 3.

A. ____________

B. ____________

C. ____________

D. ____________

A. Glomerulus

B. Proximal convoluted tubule

C. Distal convoluted tubule

D. Loop of Henle

1. Mark the following statements true or false:
   a. ______ A nephron is a tuft of capillaries which rests in the cuplike depression of Bowman's capsule.
   b. ______ Bowman's capsule and the convoluted portion of the tubule are located in the medulla of the kidney, giving it a fine, granular appearance.
   c. ______ Each kidney contains approximately one million nephrons.

1.
   a. False, this is the glomerulus
   b. False
   c. True

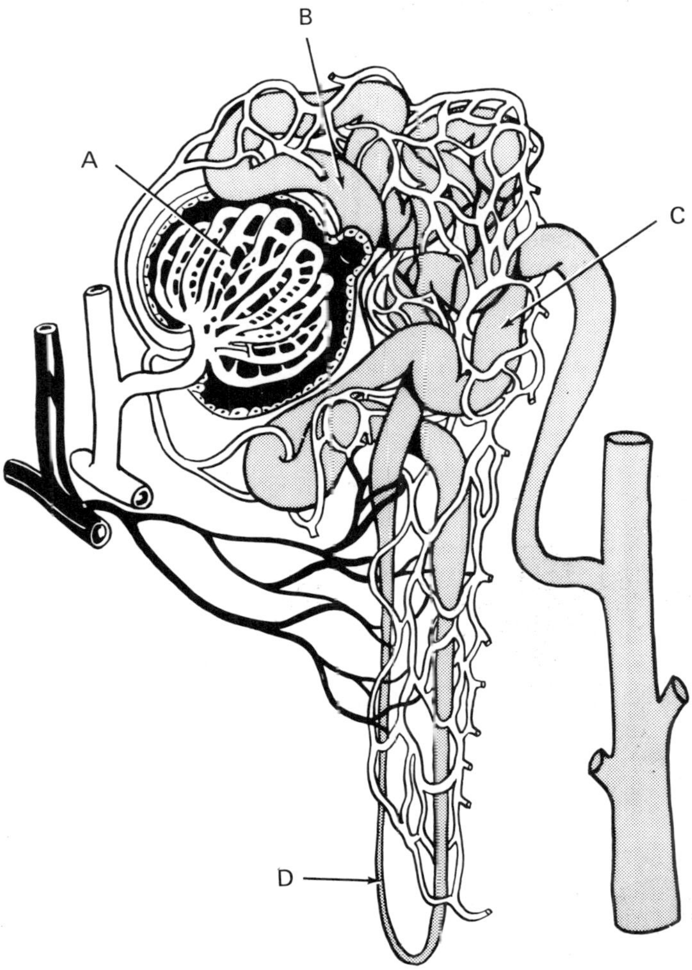


Figure 3

2. Into which of the following structures, if any, do the orifices of the collecting tubules deliver urine?

   a. Hilus
   b. Calyces
   c. Renal pelvis
   d. None of the above

2. b

3. Which of the following is commonly referred to as the functional unit of the kidney?

   a. Glomerulus
   b. Tubule
   c. Loop of Henle
   d. Nephron

3. d

4. Which vessel carries blood away from the glomerulus?

   a. Afferent arteriole
   b. Efferent arteriole
   c. Afferent venule
   d. Efferent venule

If you had any answers wrong, see Frames 8 and 9. If you were correct, go to Frame 10.

4. b

## Frame 4

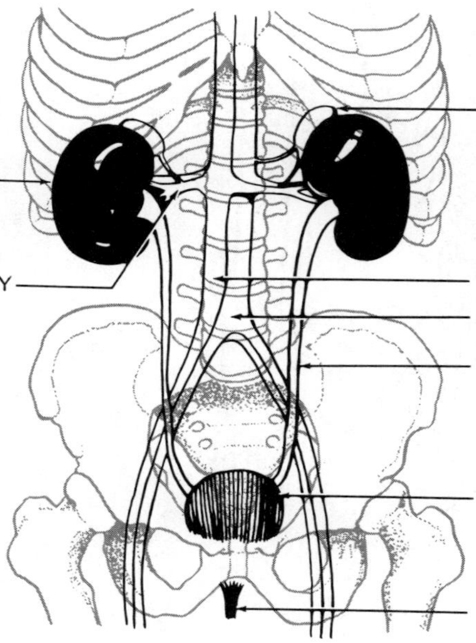


Figure 4

1. The kidneys are supplied by the __________ arteries, which branch from the __________.
2. An __________ gland lies on top of each kidney.
3. The kidneys and bladder are connected by the __________.
4. The __________ drains urine from the bladder.

1. renal
   aorta
2. adrenal
3. ureters
4. urethra

The kidneys are located in the upper (or thoracic) area of the back, and are held in place by a cushion of fat and fascia which binds them to adjacent muscles.

Return to Frame 2.

## Frame 5

Referring to the view of the renal pelvis in this figure, answer these questions:

1. Which structure is an expanded portion of the ureter?
   a. Hilus
   b. Pelvis

2. What is the function of the renal pelvis?
   a. Delivery of blood flow to the kidney
   b. Urine collection

1. b

2. b

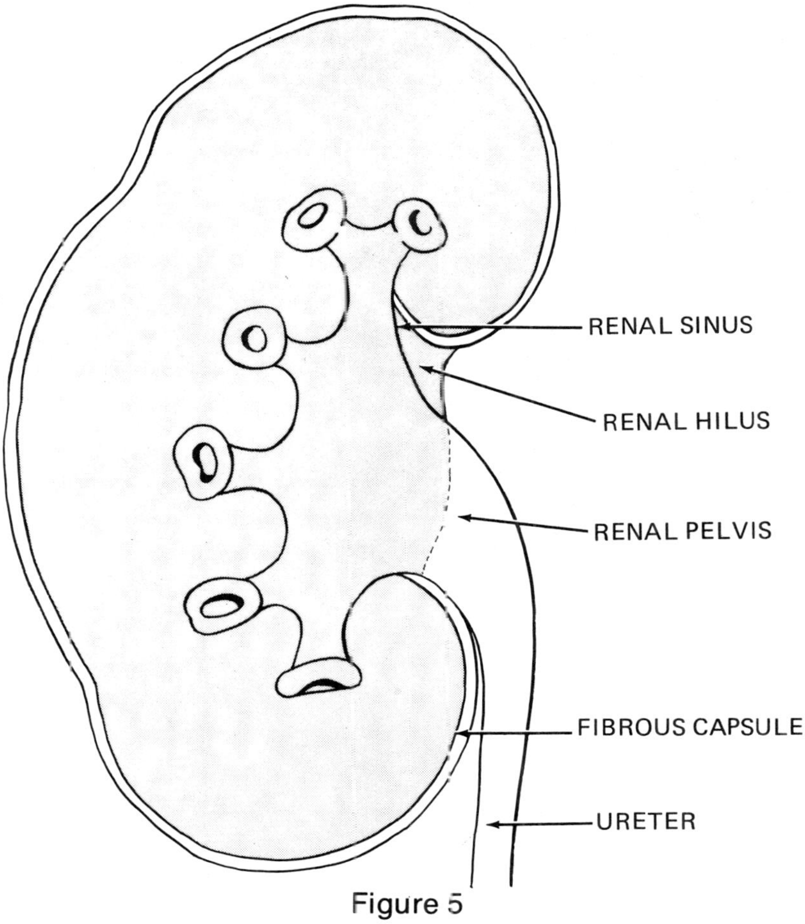


Figure 5

## Frame 6

Referring to the longitudinal section of a kidney in this figure, mark the following statements true or false:

1. ______ The large renal blood vessels divide the kidney tissue into pyramid-shaped sections.

2. ______ There is no branching of blood vessels into the cortex.

1. True

2. False

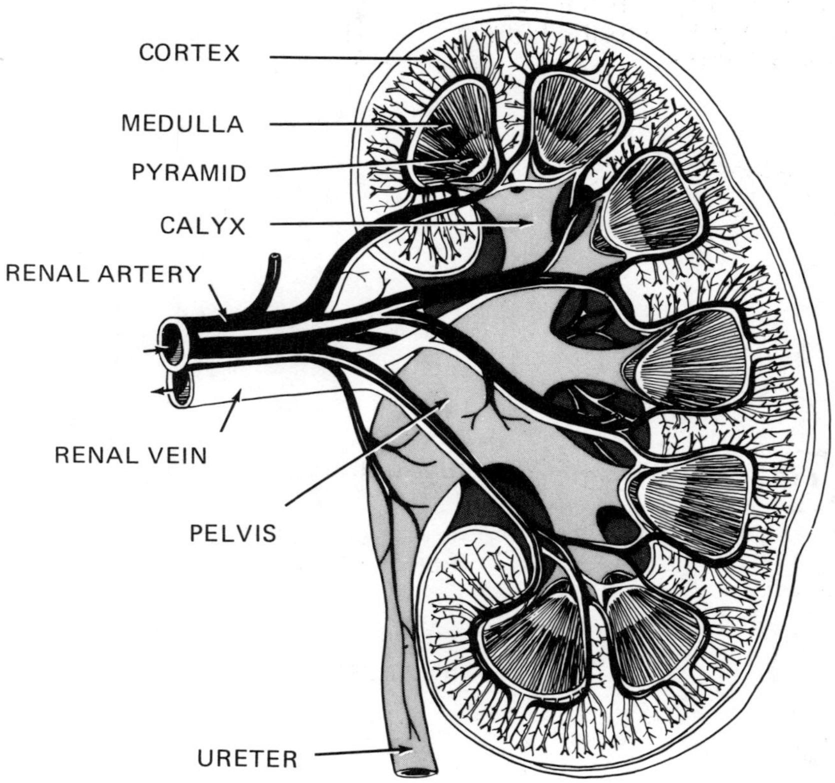


Figure 6

## Frame 7

After studying the sections of a kidney in this figure, indicate whether each of the following statements is true or false:

1. ______ The cortex contains the blood vessels and branches called glomeruli.

2. ______ The medulla contains collecting tubules.

3. ______ The collecting tubules deliver urine to the calyx.

Return to Frame 3

1. True
2. True
3. True

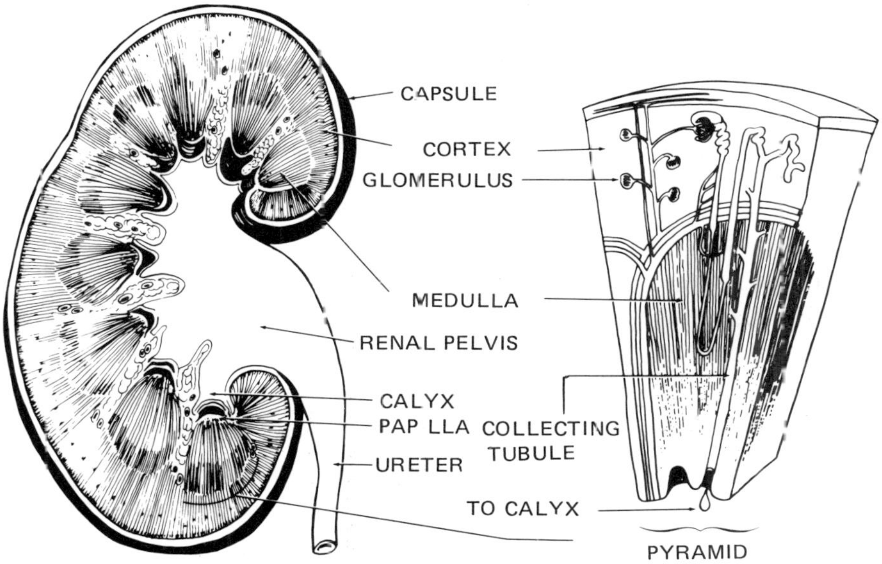


Figure 7

## Frame 8

Each kidney has about a million nephrons. The *nephron* is the functional unit of the kidney.

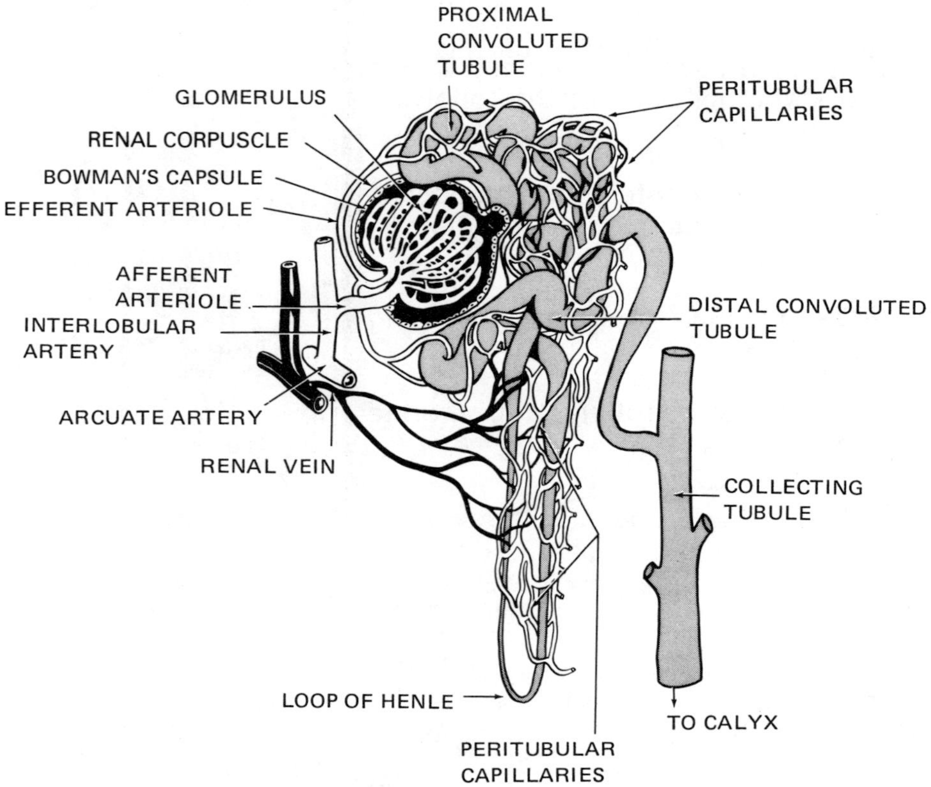


Figure 8

Trace the structures of the blood supply of the nephron shown in this figure.

1. Begin with the arcuate artery and list the structures that follow in order:

   a. ______________ ______________

   b. ______________ ______________

   c. ______________ ______________

   d. ______________ ______________

   e. ______________ ______________

   f. ______________ ______________

2. What structure is a capillary loop or tuft at the end of the afferent arteriole?

---

1.
   a. Interlobular artery
   b. Afferent arteriole
   c. Glomerulus
   d. Efferent arteriole
   e. Peritubular capillaries
   f. Renal vein

2. Glomerulus

## Frame 9

Using the figure in Frame 8, trace the kidney tubule structure of the nephron.

1. Begin with Bowman's capsule and list the structures in order.
   a.
   b.
   c.
   d.
2. What is the structure comprising the glomerulus and Bowman's capsule called?
3. What is the functional unit of the kidney called?
4. What are the two components of nephrons?
   a.
   b.

Go on to Frame 10

1.
   a. Proximal convoluted tubule
   b. Loop of Henle
   c. Distal convoluted tubule
   d. Collecting tubule
2. Corpuscle
3. Nephron
4.
   a. Glomerulus
   b. Tubules

## Frame 10

### Urine Formation

During each hour, the body's total blood volume goes through the kidneys about 12 times. The kidneys perform 2 functions vital to life:

1. Remove urea, uric acid, creatinine and other waste products from the blood to be excreted from the body
2. Regulate the composition of the blood by maintaining its water and salt concentration and acid-base balance.

Normally, an adult's kidneys filter about 170 liters of water from the blood, perform the regulating functions mentioned, and return all but about 1 or 2 liters to the bloodstream.

Mark the following statements true or false:

1. ______ The kidneys filter water from the blood and return water to the blood.

1. True

2. ______ The kidneys filter blood very slowly.

3. ______ The kidneys excrete about 1–2 liters of water and waste products each day.

2. False

3. True

## Frame 11

The filtration process takes place in the glomerulus and Bowman's capsule.

1. Blood is brought to the glomerulus by the ____________ arteriole.

2. Water and dissolved substances are filtered out of the ____________ and move into _________ _________.

3. This fluid, now called the filtrate, moves through the kidney tubules where its composition is altered by removal of ____________ and by regulation of the balance of ______________________ and ______________, and of ____________ and ____________. (Hint: see Frame 10.)

1. afferent

2. glomerulus Bowman's capsule

3. wastes water salts acids bases

## Frame 12

1. On the nephron shown in figure 9 below, shade in the location of the filtrate.

2. Now name the sections of kidney tubule indicated by the brackets.

   A.

   B.

   C.

   D.

1.

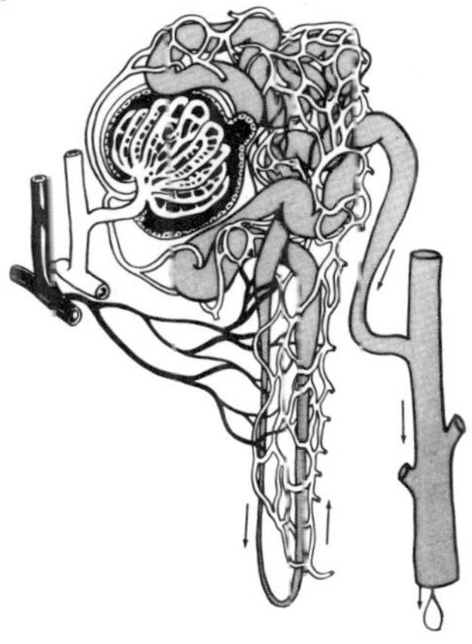

2.

A. Proximal convoluted tubule

B. Distal convoluted tubule

C. Loop of Henle

D. Collecting tubule

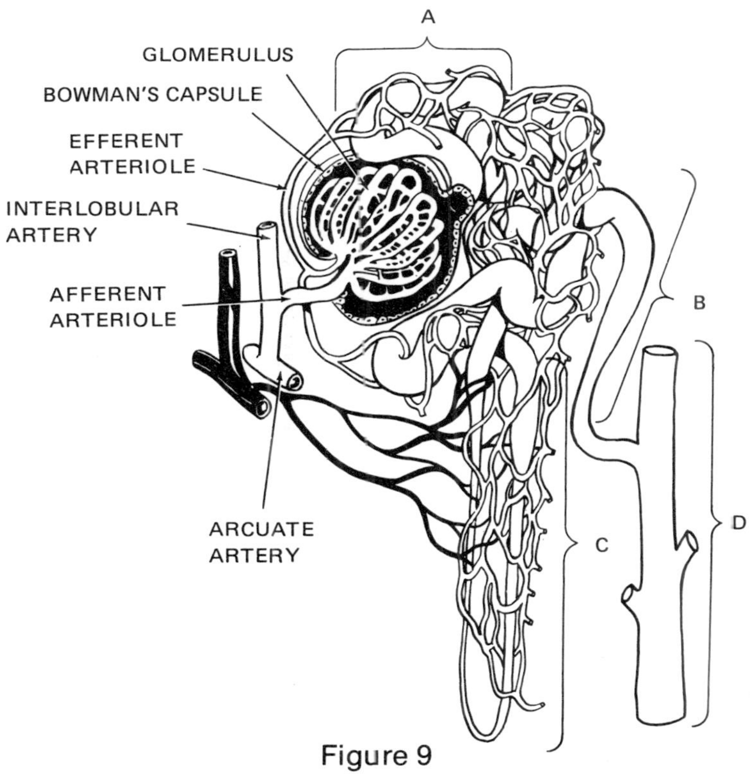


Figure 9

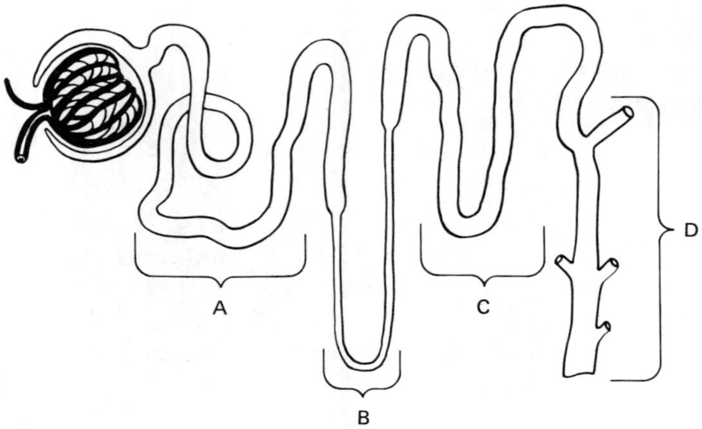


Figure 10

3. Sometimes in this book the nephron is drawn in a simplified and elongated form. Can you find each part of the tubule?

A B C D

3.

A. Proximal convoluted tubule

B. Loop of Henle

C. Distal convoluted tubule

D. Collecting duct

# CHAPTER 2

## CAUSES OF RENAL FAILURE

Many different kinds of disease processes can result in renal failure. You will see patients in critical care units who develop renal failure as a complication of their primary illness, as well as patients who are acutely ill from the effects of chronic renal failure. Early detection and prevention of renal failure are important contributions you can make. After completing this chapter you will be able to

1. Identify examples of pathologic processes that reduce blood flow and pressure in the glomerulus
2. Predict the effect of pressure changes on renal function
3. Recall the critical minimum level of systolic blood pressure needed to maintain glomerular filtration
4. Identify two kinds of antibody–antigen reactions that damage kidney tissue
5. Recognize general classifications of nephrotoxic substances
6. List three kinds of drugs that can damage the kidneys
7. Choose examples of systemic, congenital, and neoplastic diseases that affect the kidneys
8. Identify back-pressure as the damaging agent to the kidney cells in obstructive disease
9. Group the various causes of renal failure in prerenal, renal, and postrenal categories.

### Chapter outline

Prerenal causes
- Circulatory insufficiency
- Artery occlusion

Intrarenal causes
- Glomerulonephritis and autoimmune responses
- Infection
- Nephrotoxins
- Others
  - Systemic diseases
  - Polycystic disease
  - Neoplasms

Postrenal causes

# PART I
# PRERENAL CAUSES

*Panel 1*

*This was Ellen Frederick's first day as a staff nurse on the renal unit. When she arrived, the large room was quiet except for soft whirrings of machinery. Lights blinked on and off, IVs dripped. During report Ellen found out a little about the patients.*

*Mr. Jamison was transferred in from surgical ICU. Following an aortic graft he hemorrhaged and went into shock. He was taken back to surgery for repair of the graft and had produced little or no urinary output since.*

*(A detailed study of Mr. Jamison's illness will be presented in Chapter 14.)*

## Frame 1

As you can see in this figure, major arteries supply blood to the kidney. Blood is pumped

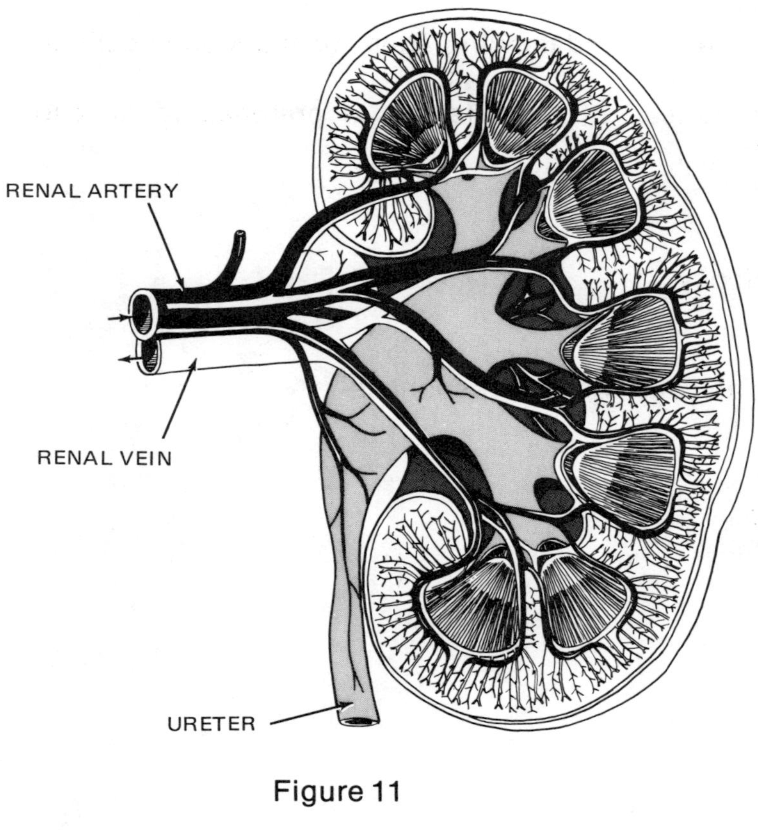


Figure 11

through this network of arteries so that the total volume of blood passes through the kidneys 12 times each hour. In order to filter this amount of blood, the kidney receives 20%–25% of the cardiac output. (Recall that the cardiac output is the amount of blood pumped out of the ventricle each minute.)

Choose the correct words in parentheses to complete the following statement:

Hemorrhagic shock implies (increased/decreased) blood volume and (increased/decreased) blood flow to the renal arteries.

decreased

decreased

## Frame 2

In Mr. Jamison's case, his low blood pressure during shock stimulated the sympathetic nervous system to adapt by:

a. Increasing the heart rate

b. Making the heartbeat more forceful

c. Constricting the blood vessels in kidneys, liver, lungs, GI tract, and skin

d. Maintaining preferential circulation to the brain and heart.

1. Which of these adaptive mechanisms would tend to get more blood to the cells?
2. Which mechanism insures blood supply for the most crucial body organs?
3. Which mechanisms are directed toward raising the blood pressure?
4. Which mechanism would decrease blood flow in the kidney?

1. a, b, d
2. d
3. a, b, c
4. c

## Frame 3

Assume that the systolic blood pressure falls below 80 mmHg due to reduced blood volume and/or low cardiac output, and the blood supply to the kidneys is severely diminished. What will happen?

1. (More/Less) blood will be filtered in the glomerulus.

1. Less

2. The urinary output will be (increased/decreased).

2. decreased

3. (More/Fewer) waste products will be removed from the blood.

3. Fewer

## Frame 4

Relating the facts about shock in Frame 3 to Mr. Jamison's case, mark the following statements true or false:

1. ______ When he was in shock, preferential circulation was given to his brain, heart, and kidneys.

1. False (not kidneys)

2. ______ Prolonged use of vasoconstricting drugs (such as levarterenol) during shock can contribute to renal failure by shutting down blood flow to the kidneys.

2. True

3. ______ If Mr. Jamison's systolic blood pressure drops below 80 mm/Hg, his kidneys will be inadequately perfused.

3. True

4. ______ Mr. Jamison's kidneys remove waste products from the blood even though no urine is produced.

4. False

## Frame 5

Diminished blood flow to the kidneys can be caused by a number of problems:

Shock

Body fluid imbalances that cause low blood volume

Poor cardiac function with less blood being pumped into the circulation

Obstruction of the renal arteries due to arteriosclerosis, stricture, or blood clots.

For each of the following disorders, fill in the blank with the letter corresponding to the mechanism by which renal blood flow is decreased:

| | | |
|---|---|---|
| 1. ______ | Renal artery thrombosis | a. Circulatory insufficiency |
| 2. ______ | Stricture of the aorta | b. Renal artery occlusion |

1. b

2. b

3. ______ Dehydration — 3. a

4. ______ Generalized arteriosclerosis — 4. b

5. ______ Severe body burn — 5. a

6. ______ Massive myocardial infarction — 6. a

**Frame 6**

The causes of renal failure are classified in different ways. One method which is easy to understand is

1. Prerenal: factors that decrease blood flow to the kidneys
2. Intrarenal: factors that directly damage kidney tissues
3. Postrenal: factors that occur in the lower urinary tract.

Shock, dehydration, burns, thrombosis of renal arteries, and arteriosclerotic vascular disease are all ____________ causes. — prerenal

**Frame 7**

Summary:

Prerenal causes of renal failure are conditions that decrease blood flow to the kidney.

If blood flow is reduced, and renal artery systolic pressure falls below 80 mm Hg, then urinary output will drop below 17 ml/hour, wastes will not be removed from the blood, and renal cells may be damaged.

Shock reduces blood flow to the kidneys. In addition, the sympathetic nervous system response of vasoconstriction of renal arteries contributes to poor perfusion of the kidneys. Other examples of disease causing circulatory insufficiency are those associated with low blood volume and/or poor cardiac output.

Other diseases classified as prerenal causes of renal failure are renal artery occlusion due to thrombosis or stricture, and narrowing of renal arteries due to arteriosclerotic disease.

# PART II
# INTRARENAL CAUSES

*Panel 2*

*Mrs. Rice was Ellen's first patient. She had a history of a strep throat infection followed by an inflammation of the kidney (glomerulonephritis). Her kidney problem had reached the stage of renal failure over a period of 15 years.*

*This type of disease is caused by the action of the immune system of the body. The body produces antibodies in protective response to the presence of bacteria, toxins or other foreign protein. The infecting organism or foreign protein is called an antigen. The body's antibodies react with the antigens and an inflammation of involved tissues results.*

*In Mrs. Rice's illness, antibodies reacted with strep-produced antigens circulating in the blood. The antigen–antibody complexes formed were trapped in the renal capillaries, causing inflammation of the filtering membranes.*

*Scientists are now intensely interested in a derangement of the immune system in which antibodies made against streptococci become "confused" and attack normal membranes of the patient's own body causing cell damage. This is called an autoimmune reaction, and it may be the cause of Mrs. Rice's continuing kidney damage.*

*(A detailed study of Mrs. Rice's illness will be presented in Chapter 11.)*

## Frame 8

Mrs. Rice had a strep infection which led to progressive direct damage to the filtering membranes of her kidneys. How would you classify this cause of renal failure? (Hint: see Frame 6)

Intrarenal cause

## Frame 9

Antibodies are formed to protect the body from the invasion of foreign proteins or antigens.

Which of the following would normally be recognized as foreign protein by antibodies?

a. Red blood cells of different blood types
b. Pathogens (germs)
c. Toxins produced by pathogens
d. A transplanted kidney
e. All of the above

e

## Frame 10

In autoimmune, or autoallergic, disease, the patient's antibodies become confused, and unable to distinguish "self" from "nonself."

1. In this kind of kidney disease, the patient's own tissues act as what?
   a. Antigens
   b. Antibodies

2. What is the result of an antigen–antibody reaction in surrounding tissue?
   a. Infection
   b. Inflammation
   c. Ischemia

3. If antigen–antibody complexes are circulating in the blood, how can they cause kidney damage?
   a. By producing poisons and toxins
   b. By being caught in the glomeruli and causing inflammation
   c. Neither, because circulating complexes are harmless

4. What pathogen frequently causes renal inflammation by its antigenic activity?

1. a
2. b
3. b
4. Streptococci

## Frame 11

Urinary tract infections are common and may be a factor in the later development of chronic renal problems. Any portion of the urinary tract may become infected: urethra, bladder, ureters or kidneys. Pyelonephritis is the infection of the kidney tissues. Organisms frequently involved are those found in the GI tract, such as *Escherichia coli* and *Enterobacter*, with ascending urinary tract infection as the mode of entry. Pathogens can also be brought to the kidney via the bloodstream in cases of sepsis.

Damage to the kidneys is caused by inflammation, fibrosis, and scarring of renal tissue. Infection tends to spread within the collecting ducts and interstitial tissue in the medulla. This slows renal blood flow and interferes with kidney function.

1. Which of the following situations could lead to pyelonephritis?
   a. Poor perineal hygiene
   b. Indwelling catheter
   c. Septicemia following a wound infection
   d. Prostatitis
   e. All of the above

1. e

2. Pyelonephritis damages the kidneys through which of the following mechanisms?
   a. Inflammation
   b. Fibrosis
   c. Scarring
   d. All of the above

2. d

## Frame 12

Just as in other parts of the body, inflammation of the filtering membranes of the kidneys can heal and leave little or no damage. Severe inflammation can, however, cause structural damage to the membranes and prevent effective filtration. The kidneys have a great reserve capacity, so the severity of the illness depends on the percent of kidney tissue affected.

True or False:

1. ______ The symptoms of renal failure get worse as a greater number of nephrons become diseased.
2. ______ The kidney has little reserve capacity.
3. ______ Infection always causes permanent structural damage to the kidneys.

1. True
2. False
3. False

## Frame 13

Inflammatory responses due to infection and immune system activity can damage the kidney tissues. However, other substances can also cause direct damage. Here is a list of renal patients who were exposed to various substances that damaged their kidneys.

Mr. Cox worked in an industrial plant where carbon tetrachloride is used.
Mrs. Simca completed a long course of gentamicin.
Mr. Harold had a complete series of x-ray diagnostic tests using contrast media containing iodine.
Mr. Garcia is a farm worker frequently exposed to insecticides.
Mrs. Wilson had taken aspirin–phenacetin–caffeine headache pills for years.
Mrs. Lind reacted to the anesthetic used in surgery.
Timmy Brown had eaten paint chips containing lead.

Choose the classes of toxic substances that can cause renal damage:

1. Whiskey
2. Industrial chemicals
3. Analgesics and anesthetics
4. Plastics
5. Heavy metals
6. X-ray dyes
7. Antibiotics

2, 3, 5, 6, 7

## Frame 14

1. How do the substances that are toxic to the kidney (nephrotoxins) come in contact with renal cells?

1. They are carried to the kidneys by the blood. (Remember: the entire blood volume goes through the kidneys 12 times each hour.)

2. Which of the substances listed in Frame 13 are related to medical treatment?

2. Antibiotics, analgesics and anesthetics, x-ray dyes

3. What are the nursing implications of use of these substances?

3. Careful observation of renal function during treatment, exact monitoring of dosage

*Panel 3*

*Here are some other diseases that directly damage kidney tissues:*

*Systemic diseases such as diabetes mellitus, lupus, and long-standing hypertension. These diseases have pathologic manifestations in the kidney, which may be due to disease of the small blood vessels or to autoimmunity. Research continues in these areas.*

*Polycystic disease. Grapelike clusters of cysts crowd out normal tissue, as shown in the figure, causing a decline in renal function. This is thought to be a genetically transmitted disease.*

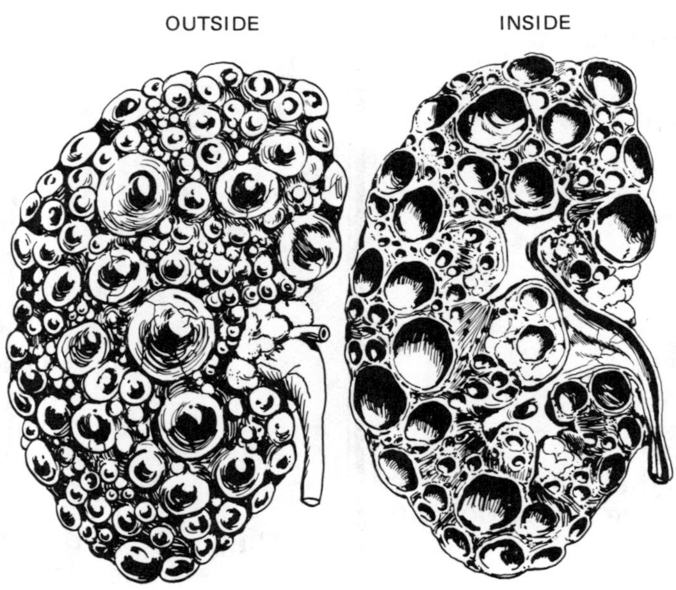


Figure 12

*Neoplastic diseases. These cause kidney problems as tumors replace normal tissue and damage other tissues by compression. Radiation treatments for cancer can also cause inflammation and damage to the kidneys.*

## Frame 15

Summary:

Intrarenal causes of renal failure are those factors that directly damage kidney tissues.

An antigen is a pathogen, toxin or tissue that is recognized by the body's immune system as foreign. Antibodies are formed to react with and destroy the antigen. The effect of this reaction on surrounding tissue is inflammation.

Frequent causes of damaging antigen–antibody reactions in the kidney are strep infections, the autoimmune response, and ascending urinary tract infections.

Some chemicals are toxic to kidney cells. Examples of these are some industrial chemicals, heavy metals, x-ray dyes, antibiotics, and analgesics.

Other intrarenal causes are systemic disease, such as diabetes mellitus, lupus, hypertension, polycystic disease, and neoplasms.

# PART III POSTRENAL CAUSES

## Frame 16

Postrenal causes of renal failure include problems of the lower urinary tract that have an effect on kidney function.

Mr. Kerry had renal stones which lodged in a ureter and blocked the flow of urine out of one kidney. This would cause (higher/lower) pressure in Bowman's capsule and the tubules. This would (help/hinder) filtration of the blood and excretion of waste products. This high back-pressure in the kidney can also lead to destruction of tissue.

higher
hinder

## Frame 17

Other conditions that cause back-pressure on the kidney tubules include any obstacle to urine flow in the lower urinary tract. Choose the examples of such problems:

a. Strictures of the ureter
b. Pelvic tumors pressing on ureters, bladder, and urethra
c. Dehydration
d. Congenital malformations of the lower urinary tract that hinder urine flow

a, b, d

## Frame 18

Summary:

Postrenal causes of renal failure are conditions such as stones, strictures, and malformations that obstruct the flow of urine out of the kidney.

The resultant back-pressure in the tubules hinders filtration of the blood and causes damage to cells.

## Frame 19

To review, the causes of renal failure may be classified as

1. Prerenal
2. Intrarenal
3. Postrenal.

Put the number of the appropriate classification after each example:

a. Autoallergic disease ______
b. Shock ______
c. Ureteral stones ______
d. Renal artery thrombosis ______
e. Severe dehydration ______
f. Burns ______
g. Polycystic disease ______
h. Renal carcinoma ______
i. Streptococcal glomerulonephritis ______
j. Exposure to nephrotoxic substance ______

a. 2
b. 1
c. 3
d. 1
e. 1
f. 1
g. 2
h. 2
i. 2
j. 2

# Section 2

# Renal Mechanisms and Their Assessment

# CHAPTER 3

## FILTRATION AND BODY PROTEIN HOMEOSTASIS

The kidney has an important part to play in the maintenance of body homeostasis. The first key function you need to understand is how the kidney filters fluid and solutes out of the blood and maintains protein balance. After completing this chapter you will be able to do the following things:

1. Identify three factors that affect filtration pressure in the glomerulus
2. Define autoregulation of glomerular filtration pressure
3. Predict the effect of damage to the glomerular membrane on filtration
4. Identify the location and extent of tubular reabsorption of protein
5. Explain the effect of glomerular osmotic pressure on filtration
6. Differentiate between anabolism and catabolism
7. Choose examples of problems related to negative protein balance
8. List two functions of the kidney in protein homeostasis
9. Predict three consequences of large losses of body protein

### Chapter outline

Pressure relationships in the glomerulus
- Filtration pressure
- Osmotic pressure
- Effective filtration pressure
- Autoregulation of renal filtration pressure

Function of the glomerular membrane
- Substances filtered
- Restriction of protein filtration
- Structure of the membrane
- Pathological problems affecting glomerular membrane function
- Systematic effects of protein loss

Protein homeostasis
- Importance of protein
- Anabolism and catabolism
- The kidney's contribution to protein homeostasis
- Systemic effects of negative protein balance

# Part I
# PRESSURE RELATIONSHIPS IN THE GLOMERULUS

## Filtration Pressure

### Frame 1

Before studying the kidney's filtering function and its role in maintaining body protein homeostasis, it is helpful to review the structure of the functional unit of the kidney, the nephron.

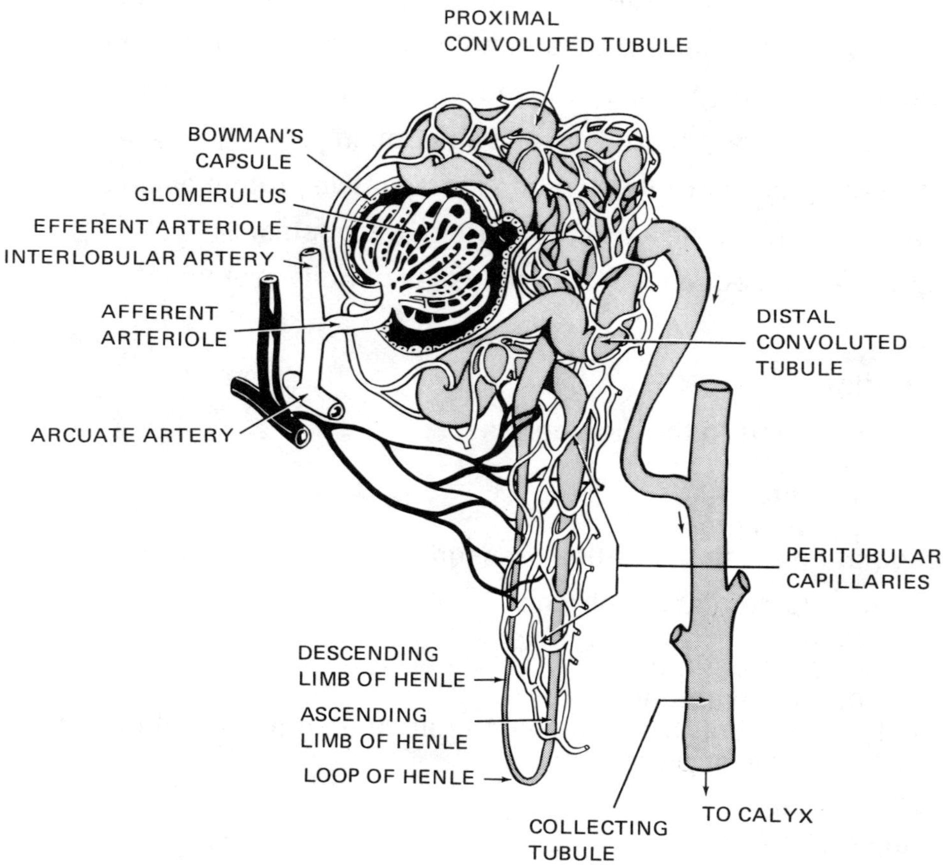


Figure 13

1. What fluid flows in the afferent arteriole and efferent arteriole? (blood/filtrate)
2. What fluid flows in the glomerulus? (blood/filtrate)
3. What fluid flows in Bowman's capsule and the proximal and distal tubules? (blood/filtrate)
4. What fluid is in the collecting duct? (blood/filtrate)

Each kidney has about a million nephrons, which all function the same way. So kidney function may be discussed in terms of one representative nephron.

1. Blood
2. Blood
3. Filtrate
4. Filtrate

## Frame 2

In order to understand how the glomerulus filters the blood, consider the example of a garden hose.

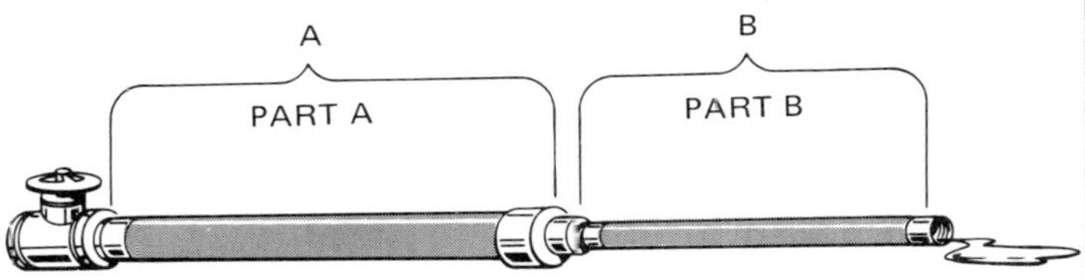


Figure 14

Referring to the figure, how would you say the smaller diameter of part B affects the water pressure in part A?

a. Makes the water pressure in A higher than if both were the same diameter
b. Makes the water pressure in A lower than if both were the same diameter
c. Does not affect the water pressure in A

a. (Because B is narrower, the outflow is obstructed. This increases pressure in A.)

## Frame 3

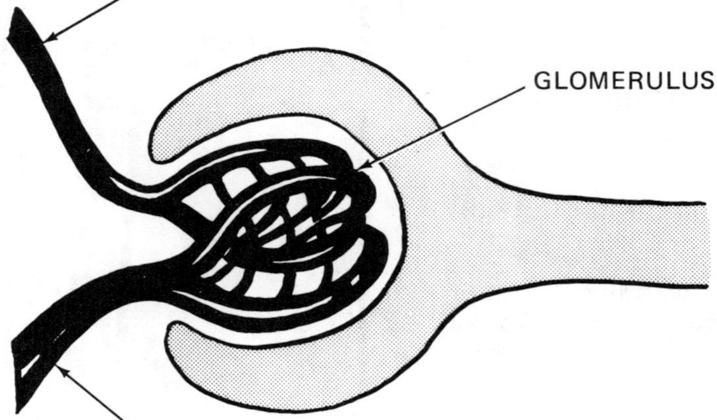


Figure 15

Look at this diagram of the glomerulus.

1. In what ways does this illustration resemble the hose in Frame 2?
   a. The afferent arteriole is like part A of the hose.
   b. The efferent arteriole is like part B of the hose.
   c. There is no relationship because the blood is flowing from efferent to afferent arterioles.
2. How does the difference in diameter between the afferent and efferent arterioles affect the blood pressure in the glomerulus? (increases/decreases)

1. a, b

2. increases

## Frame 4

The effect of the higher pressure in the glomerulus is to push fluid out of the capillaries into Bowman's capsule.

Because capillary pressure is greater than interstitial space pressure, fluid tends to flow out of the capillary.

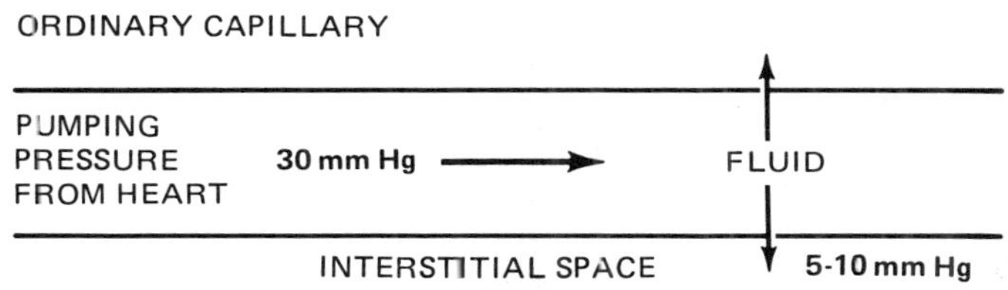


Figure 16

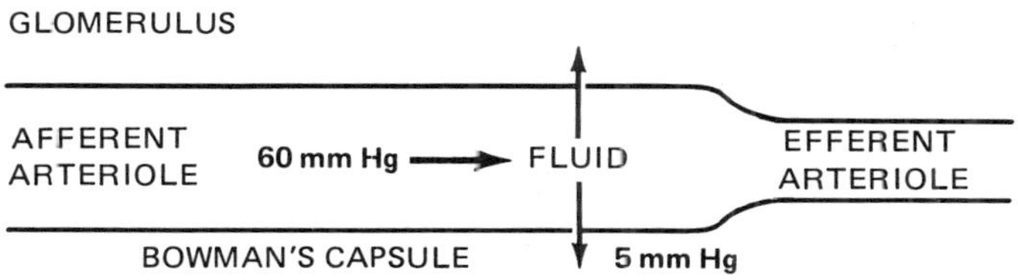


Figure 17

1. How much higher is the glomerular capillary pressure than ordinary capillary pressure?
2. The difference between fluid pressure in the capillary and the pressure in the surrounding tissue is the driving force for filtration. In which capillary would more fluid filter out?
3. Why is it advantageous for the glomerular capillary to filter more fluid out than an ordinary capillary would? (Hint: What is the purpose of the kidney?)

1. Twice as high
2. Glomerular capillary
3. So that a large portion of fluid is filtered out of the blood to be purified.

## Osmotic Pressure

### Frame 5

Osmosis is the movement of fluid across a semipermeable membrane from an area of lower to an area of higher concentration of solutes. The difference in concentration is called osmotic pressure. A semipermeable membrane is an artificial membrane such as cellophane that is permeable to fluid but not to all of the dissolved substances.

Human membranes which also allow passage of some molecules but not others are called selectively permeable. An example of this is the capillary membrane, which allows water and electrolytes to pass through, but is not permeable to protein. If there is a higher concentration of protein (and/or other substances) on one side of the membrane, water will be pulled across the membrane, tending to equalize concentrations.

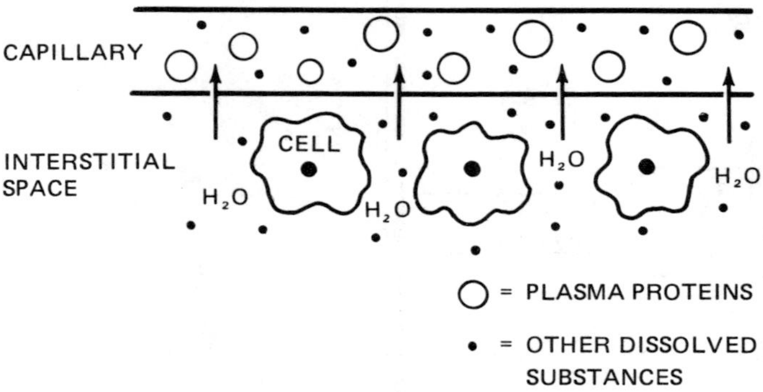


Figure 18

In this figure the higher concentration of protein and solutes in the capillary will cause water to be drawn into the capillary from the interstitial space.

1. If the blood in a capillary has a *lower* concentration of protein and electrolytes than the surrounding tissue, fluid flow will be from ____________ to ____________ ____________.

2. The osmotic pressure in the body depends on the ____________ of particles of protein and solutes on one side of a ____________ ____________ ____________.

Answers:

1. capillary
   interstitial space

2. number or concentration
   selectively permeable membrane

## Frame 6

You know that the pressure of the blood in the glomerular capillary pushes water across the capillary membrane and into Bowman's capsule. Now consider the effect of osmotic pressure. The concentration of protein and solutes is *higher* in the glomerulus than in Bowman's capsule.

1. This difference in concentration would cause water to be pulled (into/out of) the glomerular capillary.
2. This (encourages/hinders) filtration of fluid out of the blood and into the renal tubules.

Answers:

1. into
2. hinders

## Effective Filtration Pressure

### Frame 7

In the glomerulus, as noted in Frame 6, osmotic pressure works against filtration pressure.

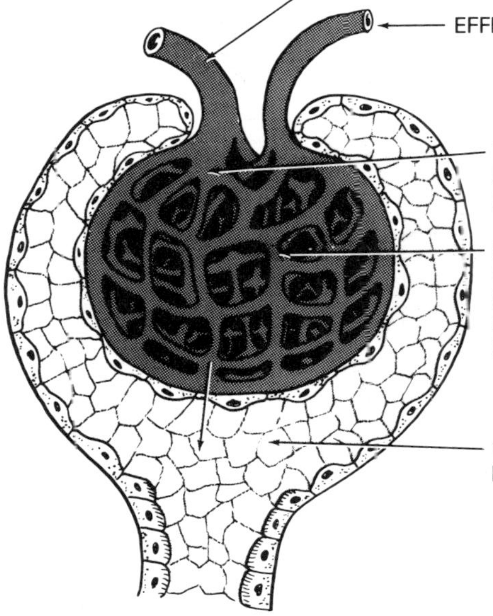


Figure 19

Using this figure, determine the amount of actual pressure driving filtration in the glomerulus.

70 mm Hg Glomerular filtration pressure

-30 mm Hg Glomerular osmotic pressure

-15 mm Hg Capsular pressure

____ mm Hg Effective filtration pressure 25

## Frame 8

Mr. Richards has a severe episode of bleeding from esophageal varices. During this time, the systolic blood pressure in his afferent arterioles is only 50 mm Hg. What effect does this have?

1. The filtration pressure of the glomerulus is (increased/decreased).
2. The effective filtration pressure is (increased/decreased).
3. The amount of filtrate presented to the tubules is (increased/decreased).

1. decreased by 20 mm Hg
2. decreased (only 5 mm Hg rather than the usual 25 mm Hg)
3. decreased

## Frame 9

Summary:

The glomerulus has a higher blood pressure than other capillaries because of the difference in diameter between inflow and outflow capillaries.

The higher filtration pressure causes fluid to move out of the glomerulus and into Bowman's capsule.

But

The higher osmotic pressure in the blood tends to prevent fluid from leaving the capillary.

The amount of actual pressure driving filtration in the glomerulus is the difference between these opposing forces.

Severe and prolonged drops in blood pressure decrease the effective filtration pressure.

## Autoregulation of Renal Filtration Pressure

## Frame 10

Under normal conditions, the blood pressure varies considerably over a 24-hour period. It is advantageous for the kidney to be able to maintain a constant filtration pressure even if the blood pressure fluctuates. For example, consider that while you are watching a monster movie, your blood pressure falls 15 mm Hg, from fright.

From what you know about the afferent and efferent arterioles, can you predict ways the kidney could maintain constant pressure?

c, d
(b could *decrease* pressure by decreasing blood flow into the glomerulus.)

a. It couldn't; pressure in the glomerulus would also fall 15 mm Hg.

b. The afferent arteriole could constrict, thus increasing pressure in the glomerulus.

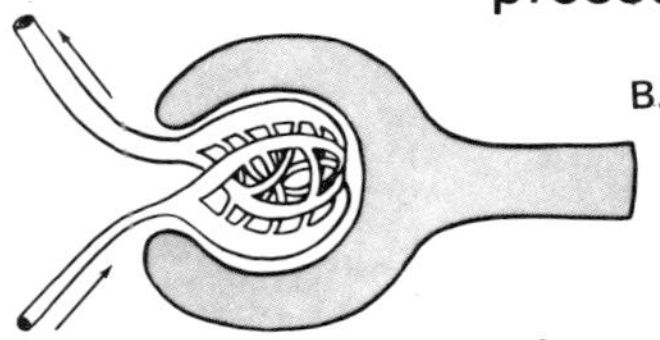

B.

c. The afferent arteriole could dilate, thus increasing pressure in the glomerulus.

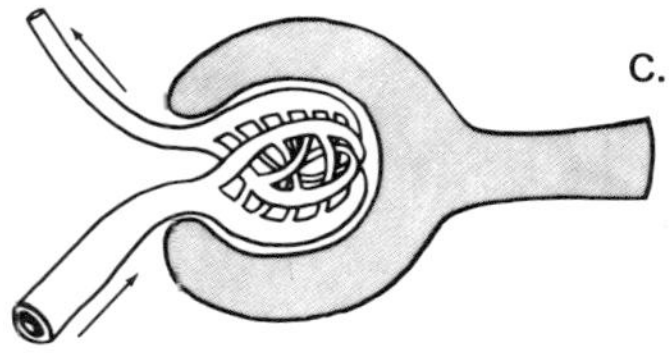

C.

d. The efferent arteriole could constrict, thus increasing pressure in the glomerulus.

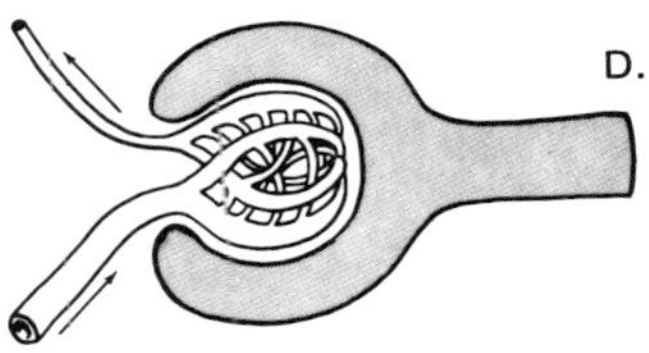

D.

Figure 20

## Frame 11

The kidney's ability to maintain a constant filtration pressure in the glomerulus, regardless of transient changes in the blood pressure, is called *autoregulation.* But, prolonged and severe changes in blood pressure and blood flow to the kidneys can cause filtration to cease.

Choose the conditions in which autoregulation would not be able to maintain glomerular filtration of blood.

a. Prolonged shock
b. Fainting
c. Blood pressure variation during sleep
d. Urinary obstruction which creates back-pressure in Bowman's capsule higher than 70 mm Hg

a, d

## Frame 12

The normal kidney will filter about 110–130 ml/min. Which of these problems would prevent the kidney from filtering this amount?

a. Loss of filtration surface in renal diseases that destroy glomeruli
b. Prolonged shock
c. Severe back-pressure due to urinary obstruction
d. Damage to the proximal and distal tubules from toxic drugs

a, b, c (The tubules are not involved in filtration.)

## Frame 13

If the kidneys are not filtering the normal amount of blood, what would the consequences be?

a. Build-up of metabolic waste products in the blood
b. Larger than normal volume of urine excreted
c. Imbalances in the amounts of acid and base in the blood

a, c

## Frame 14

What is autoregulation of filtration pressure in the glomerulus?

Autoregulation is the kidney's ability to maintain a constant filtration pressure in the glomerulus, regardless of transient changes in the systemic blood pressure. The efferent arteriole constricts, thus increasing pressure in the glomerulus.

# PART II FUNCTION OF THE GLOMERULAR MEMBRANE

## Frame 15

Now that you understand the relationship of pressure to filtration, look at another important factor, the filtering membrane.

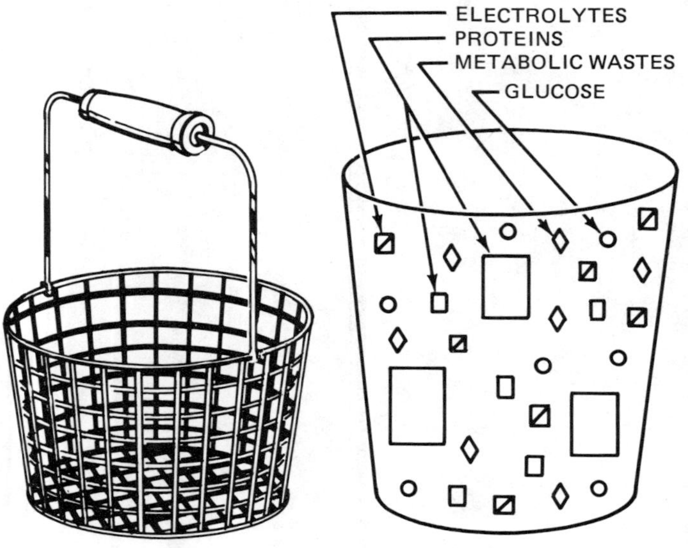


Figure 21

If the bucket of water and dissolved materials were poured into the sieve, which materials would not pass through?

Large proteins, some small proteins

## Frame 16

The wall of the glomerulus acts as a molecular sieve and keeps most of the protein and red blood cells from filtering out.

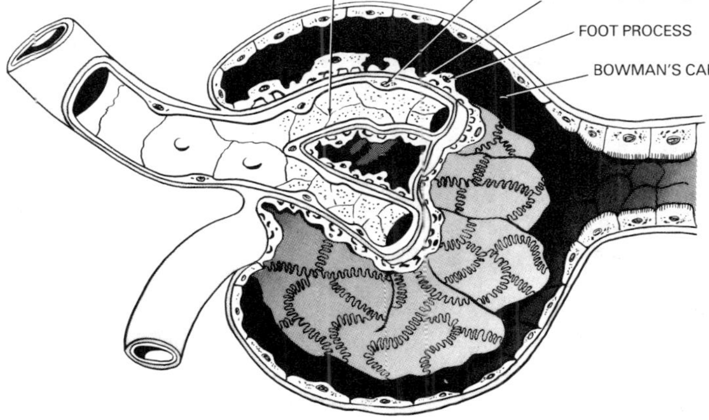


Figure 22

Examine the glomerular membrane shown in this figure. As you can see, there are three layers.

1. The layer on the inside of the capillary is the ___________ ___________. It does not constitute the barrier to protein.
2. The middle layer is called the ___________ ___________. It is composed of dense gelatinous material between two cementing layers. It is thought that the basement membrane performs the sieving function. This is also the layer that is often damaged in renal disease.
3. The outer layer is formed by epithelial cells called foot processes. This layer projects into ___________ ___________.

1. endothelial lining
2. basement membrane
3. Bowman's capsule

## Frame 17

What would happen to blood protein if the basement membrane became inflamed, widened, and more porous due to disease?

Protein would leak out into the filtrate in Bowman's capsule and then be excreted in the urine.

## Frame 18

Some small molecules of protein normally do escape the glomerular sieve, and most of these are reabsorbed by the cells lining the proximal tubule.

Decide if these statements are true or false:

1. ______ The size of a molecule determines whether it can pass through the glomerular membrane.
2. ______ Proteinuria occurs if the filtering membrane is inflamed and more porous.
3. ______ Proteinuria can occur if the tubules' capacity to reabsorb protein molecules is exceeded.

1. True
2. True
3. True

## Frame 19

Inflammation of the filtering membrane can also result in thickening and fibrosis of the membrane which blocks the filtering structure.

1. What effect would this have on filtration?
2. If a large percentage of the glomeruli were affected, what would happen to the blood's load of metabolic waste products?

1. Filtration would be hindered or stopped.
2. Waste products would be retained, and their blood levels would rise.

## Frame 20

Summary:

The glomerular membrane acts as a molecular sieve during filtration, allowing fluids, electrolytes, glucose, and waste products to be filtered out into Bowman's capsule.

Large protein molecules and red blood cells are not allowed to pass through the membrane.

Renal disease can affect the basement membrane of the glomerulus in various ways:

1. The membrane can become inflamed and more porous, allowing protein to escape into the filtrate.
2. Inflammatory processes can cause the membrane to become thick and fibrotic, preventing effective filtration of metabolic wastes.

## Frame 21

In situations where there are large losses of protein, for example, renal disease resulting in severe proteinuria, problems related to the osmotic balance of the body are seen.

Remember osmosis?

1. Draw an arrow on the figure indicating which way fluid would flow.

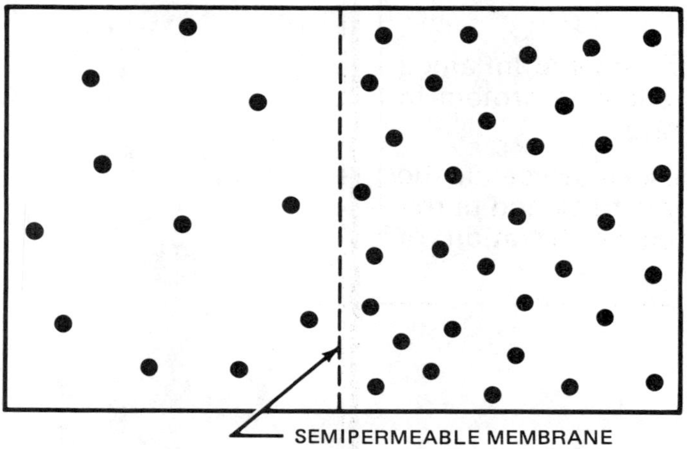


Figure 23

1.

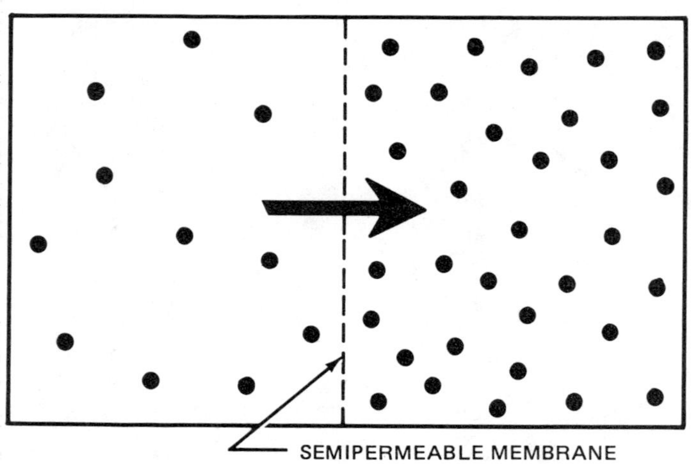

2. Osmosis refers to the flow of *fluid* across a semipermeable membrane from ______ to ______ concentration of solutes, with the effect of equalizing concentration on both sides.

2. lower
higher

**Frame 22**

If much protein is lost, for example in proteinuria, there is a lower concentration of protein in the plasma.

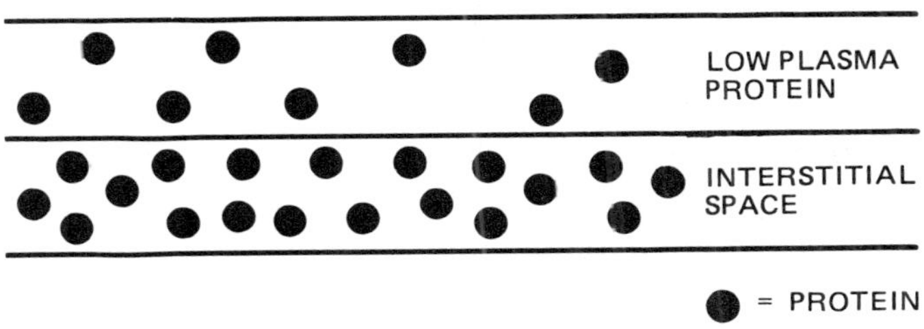


Figure 24

1. Indicate on the figure above which way fluid would flow.

1. Out of the blood and into the interstitial space

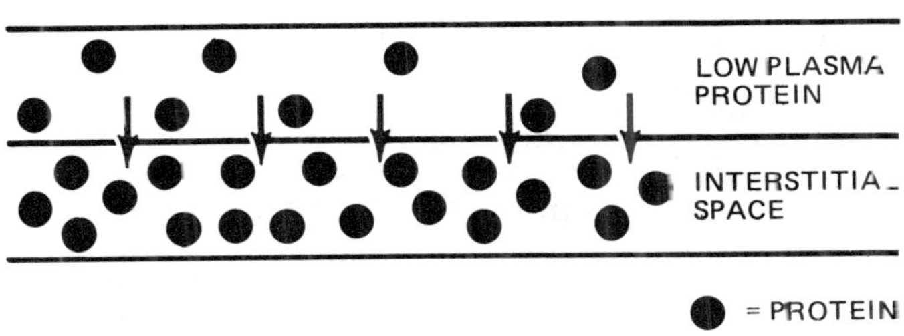


2. Excess fluid in the interstitial space is called ______.

2. edema

# PART III
# PROTEIN HOMEOSTASIS

## Frame 23

The kidney's role in protein homeostasis is important because protein stands at the very center of life by forming the basic structure of all cells and of enzymes. In addition, protein can supply energy in combination with other compounds. Amino acids are combined chemically to form various proteins.

Structural elements of the cells are not fixed and stable—rather they are constantly undergoing a regulated tearing down and resynthesis, requiring new amino acids for the process.

Mark the following statements true or false:

1. _____ Every cell in the body is continually renewing its components.
2. _____ Protein is a building-block material, not an energy source.
3. _____ Enzymes are made out of protein.
4. _____ Regular intake of protein is not necessary as protein renews itself in the body.

1. True
2. False
3. True
4. False

## Frame 24

The growth and repair of body protein, and assimilation of amino acids for this constructive process is called *anabolism.*

The release of energy by oxidation of organic foods is called *catabolism.*

Mark these statements true or false:

1. _____ In the normal, healthy adult, anabolism and catabolism are in balance.
2. _____ Amino acids are used in the body to build cells.
3. _____ Rebuilding cellular structures is an example of catabolism.
4. _____ Burning muscle protein for energy is an example of anabolism.

1. True
2. True
3. False
4. False

## Frame 25

Now look at what happens to amino acids (the building blocks used to form protein) when they are absorbed from the GI tract.

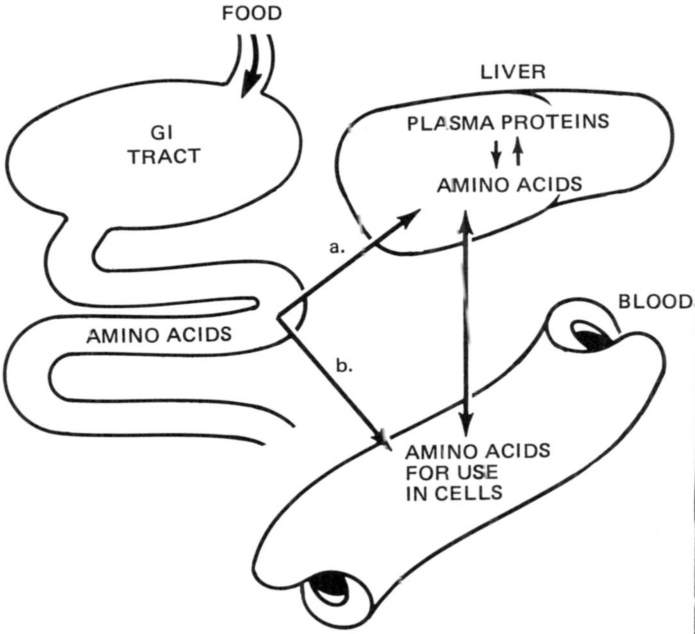


Figure 25

Fill in the blanks, noting what happens at locations a and b in the figure:

a. Amino acids are carried to the ________ to be made into ________ ________________.

liver
plasma protein

b. They are delivered by the blood stream to ______________.

cells

## Frame 26

The liver uses amino acids to synthesize new plasma protein, when needed, to keep the blood level in the normal range and maintain osmotic pressure. Enough amino acids must be available in the blood for this process to continue.

If the blood supply of amino acids is low, and more are needed by the cells, the liver can change plasma protein back to amino acids for use by the cells.

Mark the statements true or false:

1. ______ Starvation would decrease amino acids in the blood.
2. ______ Plasma protein functions as a backup supply of amino acids for the cells.
3. ______ The liver synthesizes plasma protein at a fixed rate.

1. True
2. True
3. False (The rate varies according to the blood level of protein.)

## Frame 27

Once amino acids are delivered to the cells they are used to build cellular protein. If needed, they can also be oxidized for energy.

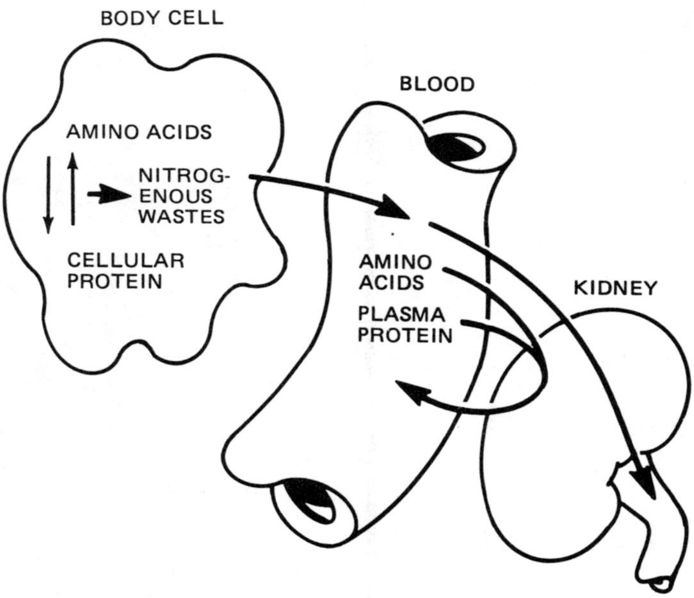


Figure 26

1. What are the by-products of protein utilization in the cells?
2. Complete the following sentences describing the two functions of the kidney in maintaining protein homeostasis?
   a. Nitrogenous wastes are ______________.
   b. Amino acids and plasma protein are __________.

1. Nitrogenous wastes (urea, uric acid, creatinine)
2.
   a. excreted
   b. saved

## Frame 28

If a patient uses or loses more protein than he takes in, he is in negative protein balance.

This can be caused by

Deficiencies in intake, absorption, and synthesis of protein by the liver

Excessive losses in urine, infection, drainage, trauma.

1. Choose the conditions which could result in negative protein balance:
   a. Starvation
   b. Profuse wound drainage
   c. Severe hepatitis
   d. Proteinuria
   e. Diseases affecting absorption from the GI tract
   f. Extensive burns
   g. All of the above

1. g

2. What effects do you think negative protein balance would have on the body? (Hint: review frame 23.)

2. Decreased growth and repair of cells, less metabolic efficiency due to lack of materials for enzymes, less capacity for energy production, inability to manufacture enough hemoglobin

## Frame 29

Ellen's patient, Mrs. Rice, had glomerulonephritis caused by strep infection and damage to the glomerular membranes. She had 4+ proteinuria and a low plasma protein level.

Mark these statements true or false:

1. ______ The low plasma protein reflects the liver's inability to make up for large urinary losses of protein.

1. True

2. ______ Loss of protein in the urine does not change the osmotic pressure in the blood.

3. ______ If the osmotic pressure in the blood decreases, fluid will move out of the blood into the interstitial space.

4. ______ Mrs. Rice would be edematous because of osmotic factors.

2. False

3. True

4. True

## Frame 30

If you had trouble with Frame 29, continue with this frame.

A patient who is losing large amounts of protein in the urine may have lower plasma protein because the cells' need for amino acids continues unabated. The plasma protein is utilized for this purpose, and the liver may be unable to keep up with the demands for new plasma protein.

If the plasma protein level is low, fluid will move from the blood vessels to the interstitial space by osmosis.

Excess fluid in the interstitial space is called edema.

## Frame 31

Summary:

Anabolism is the building up and repair of body protein through absorption of amino acids and synthesis of these into protein.

Catabolism is the release of energy by oxidation of organic foods.

These two processes are in balance in the healthy adult.

If more protein is lost than is taken in by the body

1. Negative protein balance occurs, with decreased metabolic efficiency and lack of repair of cells
2. The osmotic pressure of the blood is lessened, resulting in edema.

The two main functions of the kidney in maintaining protein homeostasis are

1. To excrete the by-products of protein metabolism
2. To prevent loss (urinary excretion) of protein and amino acids.

# CHAPTER 4

# ASSESSMENT: BODY PROTEIN HOMEOSTASIS

A number of clinical laboratory tests of blood and urine give valuable information about the kidneys' ability to maintain protein homeostasis. Problems with this function also cause distinctive physical symptoms.

At the completion of this chapter you will be able to

1. Differentiate between qualitative and quantitative measurements of proteinuria
2. Recognize the level of proteinuria indicating renal disease
3. Relate serum albumin levels to decreased intake or urinary loss of protein
4. Recognize symptoms occurring in the nephrotic syndrome
5. Relate symptoms of nephrotic syndrome to causes.

## Chapter outline

Urinalysis
- Quantitative
- Qualitative

Blood protein

Nephrotic syndrome

# PART I URINALYSIS

## Frame 1

In Chapter 3 you learned that damage to the glomerular sieve can disrupt protein homeostasis. The effects of this can be evaluated by noting the amount of protein in blood and urine and by observing the patient's physical symptoms.

The protein measured in a 24-hour urine collection is usually albumin because it is a small molecule and is more easily lost. Normal excretion would be in the range of 40–80 mg, but can reach 150 mg daily.

1. Proteinuria usually indicates (glomerular/tubular) damage.

1. glomerular (If you answered tubular, turn back and review the section on the glomerular sieve in Chapter 3.)

2. The level of proteinuria indicating damage would be any level greater than (80 mg daily/150 mg daily).

2. 150 mg daily

## Frame 2

A urine specimen can be analyzed to find the quantity and quality of its elements. A 24-hour urine collection is needed to find the number of milligrams or grams of protein lost in the urine. This is a *quantitative* test and is an accurate measurement of protein lost.

A test to show merely the presence or absence of various constituents of urine is called a *qualitative* test. A routine urinalysis will indicate the presence of protein on a scale of 0 to 4+. This is a rough index, and a quantitative test is needed to find out exactly how much protein is lost.

1. Indicate whether each of these lab reports is a qualitative or quantitative measurement:
   a. A lab report of 150 mg albumin in a urine specimen
   b. A lab report of 3+ albumin in a urine specimen

1.
   a. Quantitative
   b. Qualitative

2. Which type of measurement is more accurate?

2. Quantitative (measures actual amount)

3. Which type of measurement would be useful in screening a large number of patients for abnormalities in the urine?

3. Qualitative (quickly identifies whether protein is in the urine)

## Frame 3

For a month Jo Smith has had more than 3 g protein in 24-hour urine collections.

What does Jo's continuous proteinuria indicate about her kidneys?

There is damage to ______________.

glomerular membranes

# PART II
# BLOOD PROTEIN

## Frame 4

A normal serum albumin level is 3.2–5.6 g/100 ml. The principal function of albumin is to provide colloid osmotic pressure in the blood. The serum albumin level will be lowered if albumin is lost in the urine.

1. A high *urine* albumin level would be associated with a (high/low) *serum* level.
2. Jo Smith is excreting greater than 3 g albumin. Her serum albumin level would most likely be (4.2 g/2.2 g).
3. Jo will have (high/low) capillary osmotic pressure, causing fluid to move (into/out of) the capillaries.

1. low
2. 2.2g
3. low, out of

## Frame 5

Globulin and fibrinogen are two other major blood proteins. Globulins are primarily responsible for forming natural and acquired immunity. Fibrinogen is involved in making fibrin which is necessary for blood clotting.

Since the person with renal failure may have decreased levels of these proteins due to a protein restricted diet, poor dietary intake, or urinary loss, what results could you expect?

1. The person with renal failure will have an (increased/decreased) immunity to infection.
2. Clotting occurs (quickly/slowly) when kidney failure is present.

1. decreased
2. slowly

## Frame 6

Hemoglobin is made from protein and iron. When the pool of body protein is low, fewer red blood cells can be formed. The result of this is anemia.

The normal hemoglobin level is
Men: 14–18 g/100 ml
Women: 12–16 g/100 ml

1. Would Jo Smith, who is becoming protein-depleted, probably have a hemoglobin level above or below 12 g/100 ml?

Below

# PART III
# NEPHROTIC SYNDROME

## Frame 7

Jo Smith's illness is an example of glomerular disease causing large protein loss and edema. All of the symptoms associated with this condition are called the nephrotic syndrome.

1. Jo's serum albumin—less than 1 g/100 ml—is due to urinary (loss/gain).
2. This (increases/decreases) the protein concentration in the blood.
3. The change in protein concentration (raises/lowers) osmotic pressure in the blood.
4. Fluid will (leave/go to) the interstitial space.

1. loss
2. decreases
3. lowers
4. go to

## Frame 8

If the nephrotic syndrome continues unchecked, there will be evidence of protein malnutrition. Why would this be so?

1. Protein loss would be (greater/less) than dietary intake of protein.
2. The depleted protein means use of body stores for energy. This is (catabolism/anabolism).
3. When protein use or loss is greater than its intake, (negative/positive) nitrogen balance exists in the body.

1. greater
2. catabolism (For review see Chapter 3, Frame 24.)
3. negative (For review see Chapter 3, Frame 28.)

## Frame 9

Mr. Casey is brought to the ICU following a cardiac arrest on the nephrology station. He was admitted for nephrotic syndrome associated with hypertensive renal vascular disease.

In assessing Mr. Casey's renal function, what symptoms would you expect that are related to protein homeostasis?

1. Urinalysis: ____________
2. Serum albumin: ____________
3. Shifts in body fluid: from ____________ to ____________

1. proteinuria
2. low, less than 2.0 g/100 ml
3. plasma
interstitial space

## Frame 10

Summary:

Assessment parameters for body protein homeostasis are

Urinalysis

Quantitative: measurement of the amount of protein in the urine
Qualitative: presence or absence of protein in urine, 0 to 4+ scale

Serum albumin levels

Normal: 3.2–5.6 g/100 ml
Decreases if protein is excreted in urine or if protein intake is poor

Physical symptoms of low serum albumin

Edema due to decreased plasma osmotic pressure
Protein malnutrition

Hemoglobin levels
Normal
Men: 14–18 g/100 ml
Women: 12–16 g/100 ml

Depletion of globulin causes decreased resistance to disease.

Low fibrinogen levels are associated with slow blood clotting.

Low hemoglobin causes symptoms of anemia.

# CHAPTER 5

## RENAL MECHANISMS: REABSORPTION AND EXCRETION OF SOLUTES

In the previous chapters you reviewed the filtration process in the glomeruli. Each minute approximately 600 ml plasma flows through the kidneys, and of this about 120 ml is filtered out. The kidney tubules then reabsorb substances needed by the body and excrete unneeded and toxic substances. The "sorting out" process is the subject of this chapter.

After finishing this chapter you will be able to

1. Identify which substances are excreted and reabsorbed by the kidney tubules
2. Define threshold and give an example of a threshold substance
3. Explain the following facts about sodium, calcium, phosphorus and potassium:
    a. Importance in the body
    b. Control of mechanisms
    c. Kidney regulation
    d. Effects of kidney disease

### Chapter outline

Filtration, reabsorption and excretion
- Threshold substances
- Waste products of metabolism

Electrolytes
- Sodium
    - Importance in the body
    - Location of reabsorption
    - Control mechanisms
    - Effect of kidney disease
- Calcium and Phosphorus
    - Balance between serum and bone
    - Control mechanisms
    - Kidney regulation
    - Effect of kidney disease
- Potassium
    - Mechanisms of excretion
    - Effects of imbalances

# PART I FILTRATION, REABSORPTION, AND EXCRETION

## Frame 1

The tubules reabsorb 70%–80% of the glomerular filtrate. This table shows the amount of each substance filtered out of the blood and the amount that is finally excreted in a 24-hour period.

**Table 1**
**Substances Filtered out of the Blood and Excreted in a 24-hour Period**

| Substance | Amount in filtrate | Amount in urine | Percent not reabsorbed |
|---|---|---|---|
| Sodium | 600 g | 6 g | 1 |
| Potassium | 35 g | 2 g | 6 |
| Calcium | 5 g | 0.2 g | 2.2 |
| Glucose | 200 g | 0 | 0 |
| Urea | 60 g | 35 g | 65 |
| Water | 180 liters | 1.5 liters | 0.9 |
| Amino acids | 10 g | 300 mg | 3 |

Geschickter, Charles F. and Tatiana Antonovych, *The Kidney in Health and Disease* (Philadelphia: J.B. Lippincott, 1971, p. 11)

1. List the substances in order, according to *how completely* they are *reabsorbed* from the filtrate. Begin with the highest reabsorption.
   a.
   b.
   c.
   d.
   e.
   f.
   g.

1.
a. Glucose
b. Water
c. Sodium
d. Calcium
e. Amino acids
f. Potassium
g. Urea

2. What would happen to the body if 99% of the water were not reabsorbed each day?

2. Dehydration resulting in death

3. Which of the substances listed is an abnormal constituent of urine?

3. Glucose

## Frame 2

The nitrogenous waste products of protein metabolism are also filtered from the blood.

*Urea* is the major end product of protein metabolism that is excreted by the kidney. Some of the urea is reabsorbed and utilized to make protein. The kidney excretes about 35% of the urea, depending on the amount of urine formed. The concentration of urea in the interstitial space of the kidney influences the concentration and dilution of the urine.

*Creatinine* is a waste product from muscle protein metabolism. It is almost completely filtered from the blood and excreted.

1. If you wanted to study the ability of the kidneys to completely filter and excrete nitrogenous wastes, which of these substances would you measure in blood and urine? (urea/creatinine)

1. Creatinine (It is almost completely filtered from the urine.)

*Ammonia* is also formed from waste nitrogen. It is excreted by the kidney as part of the body buffering process.

Other compounds are also completely excreted by the kidneys such as dyes, medicines, and toxic materials.

Mark this statement true or false:

2. ______ If the kidney were not able to excrete the normal level of nitrogenous wastes, the serum levels of urea and creatinine would rise.

2. True

## Frame 3

The kidney uses

*Osmosis:* To reabsorb water
*Diffusion* and
*Active transport:* To reabsorb solutes

Quickly review these ideas:

Diffusion is the movement of dissolved substances from an area of higher to an area of lower concentration. The difference in concentrations is called a gradient. Consider the following examples:

If a tablet of salt is put in the bottom of a glass of water, as shown in the figure, the salt molecules will move throughout the solution until they are equally distributed.

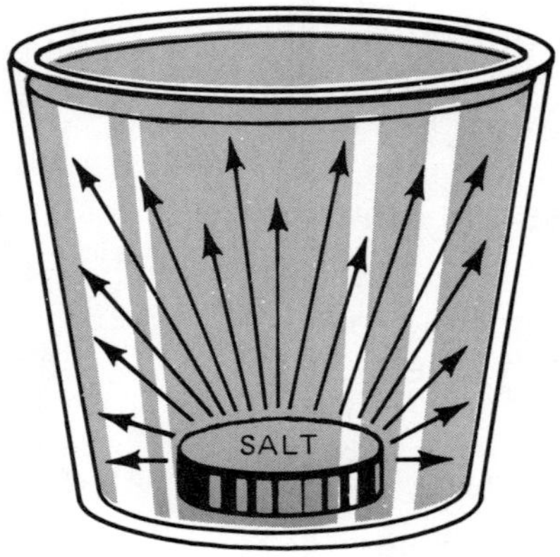


Figure 27

If two solutions are separated by a membrane that is permeable to a dissolved substance, as exemplified by the capillary in this figure, the substance will cross the membrane until concentrations on both sides are equal.

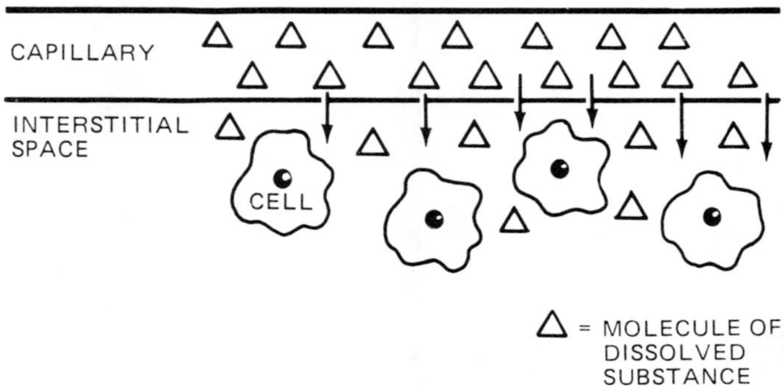


Figure 28

An electric gradient can also be created. In a container with a substance carrying a positive charge on one side of a membrane permeable to the chemicals, and a substance carrying a negative charge on the other side, as shown in the figure, the chemicals would move to equalize the charges.

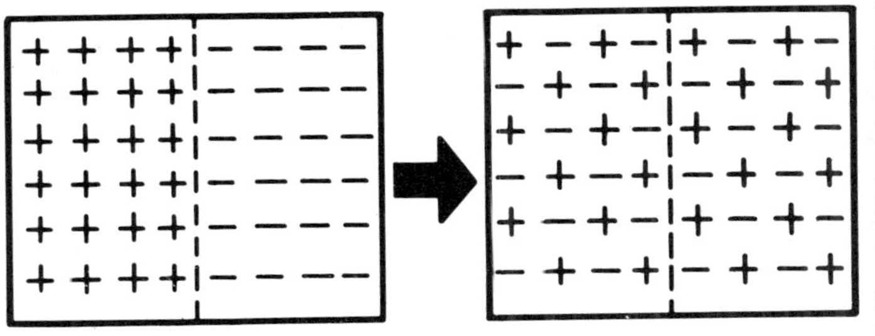

Figure 29

1. In this figure, make an arrow to show the direction of movement of △ (a solute molecule).

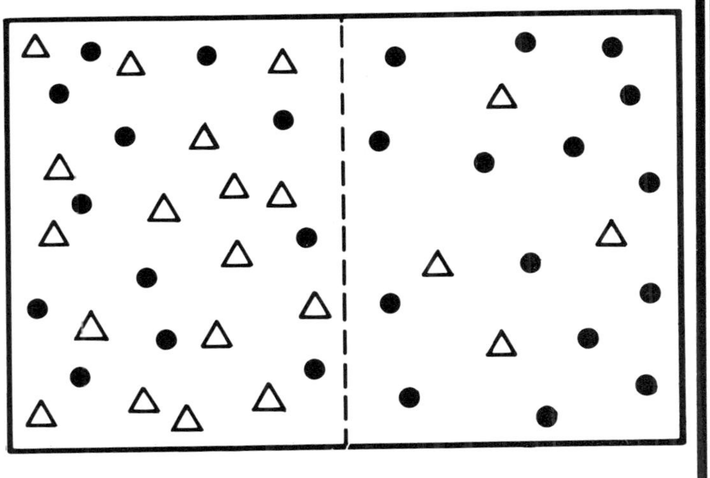

Figure 30

1. 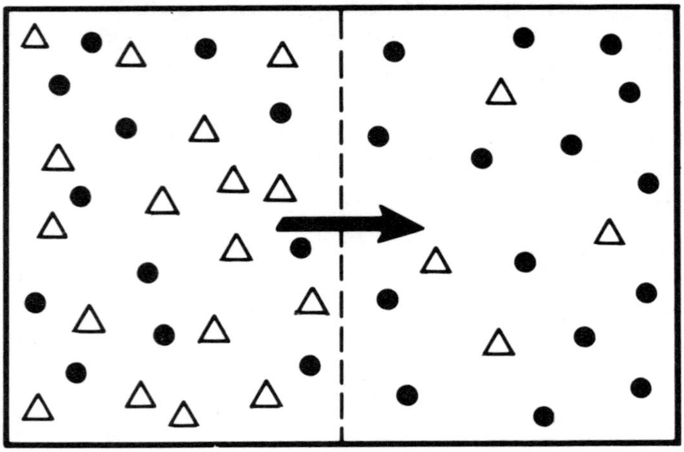

2. Choose the ways in which diffusion differs from osmosis. (Hint: You may need to review osmosis in Chapter 3, Frame 5)
   a. The fluids move in diffusion.
   b. The membrane is permeable to the solute in diffusion.
   c. In osmosis, fluid flow is from lesser to greater concentration of solutes.

b, c

## Frame 4

Active transport is the movement of dissolved substances *against* concentration and electric gradients.

For example: consider the kidney tubule starting to reabsorb glucose ($\Delta$) in part A of this figure. Here glucose can move along a concentration gradient.

Later, as may be seen in part B of this figure, the concentration of glucose is equal on both sides of the tubular membrane. Diffusion is completed, and much glucose would be excreted and wasted, if it were not for another process.

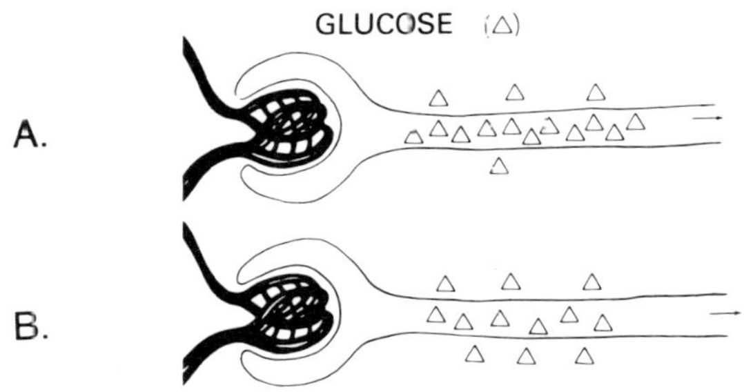


Figure 31

The tubules should reabsorb *all* of the glucose.

This is done by means of carriers which use metabolic energy to move the glucose across the membrane *against* the gradient.

Active transport involves which of these factors?

a. Expenditure of energy
b. Dependence on diffusion gradients
c. Special carrier molecules
d. Movement against diffusion gradients

a, c, d (b is wrong because active transport does not depend on diffusion gradients at all.)

## Frame 5

Match the terms on the left with the definitions on the right.

| | |
|---|---|
| 1. Osmosis | a. Substances are moved across membranes against concentration and electric gradients by carrier molecules. |
| 2. Diffusion | b. Fluid moves across a semipermeable membrane from an area of lesser concentration of solutes to an area of greater concentration. |
| 3. Active transport | c. Dissolved substances move from an area of higher to lower concentration. |

1. b
2. c
3. a

## Frame 6

Now look more closely at the process of reabsorption of useful substances in the filtrate. Some of the solutes diffuse out of the filtrate in accord with their chemical or electric gradients. However, many of the solutes are transferred in or out of the tubules by active transport. One way the body regulates reabsorption involves a concept called threshold.

Threshold substances are

Useful to the body (Examples include glucose, amino acids, sodium, chloride, and phosphorus.)

Reabsorbed in different amounts, according to the normal plasma levels of the substance.

Nonthreshold substances are

Not useful to the body (Examples include creatinine and toxins.)

Are not selectively reabsorbed, but a small amount may diffuse back into the blood from the tubules.

True or False:

1. _____ A threshold substance is reabsorbed from the filtrate in amounts needed to maintain normal plasma levels of that substance.
2. _____ Creatinine is an example of a threshold substance.
3. _____ The amount of a nonthreshold substance will be higher in urine than in plasma, as it is not reabsorbed by the tubules.

1. True
2. False (Most creatinine is excreted.)
3. True

## Frame 7

Most of the threshold substances have a "tubular maximum," which is the maximum ability of the tubule to actively reabsorb the substance in order to replenish the blood level. Any excess substance is excreted.

Mrs. Kaiser has a serum glucose level of 220 mg/100 ml (normal: 60–100 mg/100 ml). She also has glucose in her urine.

1. Glucose (is/is not) a threshold substance.
2. There is a (higher/lower) than normal amount of glucose in Mrs. Kaiser's plasma and glomerular filtrate.
3. This glucose level is (greater/less) than the tubule's reabsorptive capacity.
4. The excess glucose is (reabsorbed/ excreted).

Answers:

1. is
2. higher
3. greater
4. excreted

## Frame 8

Summary:

Substances that are almost completely reabsorbed from the urinary filtrate are water, glucose, sodium, calcium, and amino acids.

Substances that are largely excreted by the kidneys are nitrogenous wastes (urea, creatinine), toxins, dyes, and other compounds not useful to the body.

One method by which the body regulates reabsorption is through a threshold mechanism. Threshold substances are reabsorbed from the filtrate in amounts needed to keep serum levels within normal limits.

# PART II ELECTROLYTES

## SODIUM

### Frame 9

Now consider how some of the major electrolytes are reabsorbed by the tubules and how this process is affected by renal disease. Begin with sodium (Na).

Sodium is an important substance, as it is the chief extracellular ion. Therefore, the kidneys reabsorb most of it to precisely maintain sodium balance. Since water follows sodium in the body, the fluid balance of the body is also closely linked to this process.

This figure shows where sodium is removed from the filtrate by means of active transport, and where the hormone aldosterone acts to further conserve sodium.

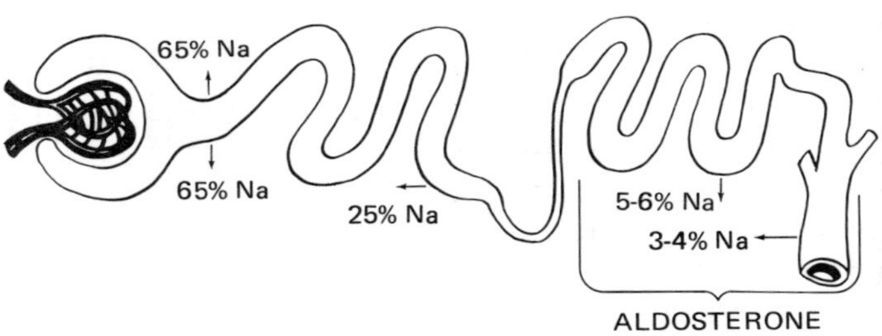


Figure 32

True or false:

1. ______ Most of the sodium in the filtrate is reabsorbed by the proximal tubule.
2. ______ Aldosterone affects sodium reabsorption in the distal tubule.

1. True
2. True

### Frame 10

1. Is it correct to say that the chief objective of tubular action on sodium is to conserve it?
2. What hormone is influential in regulating sodium reabsorption?

1. Yes
2. Aldosterone

*Panel 1*

*There are a number of factors that influence the amount of sodium that is reabsorbed. The major factors are*

1. Glomerular Filtration Rate. *If filtration is increased, the amount of sodium filtered also increases. In an effort to save sodium, tubular reabsorption also increases.*
2. Aldosterone. *The kidney's regulation of sodium is closely allied to extracellular fluid volume, so tubular reabsorption must be sensitive to changes in the fluid volume of the blood and interstitial space. This is accomplished by the juxtaglomerular (JG) system. As you can see in the figure, the distal tubule lies close to the glomerulus.*

*Special JG cells in and around the distal tubule sense perfusion pressure in the afferent arteriole.*

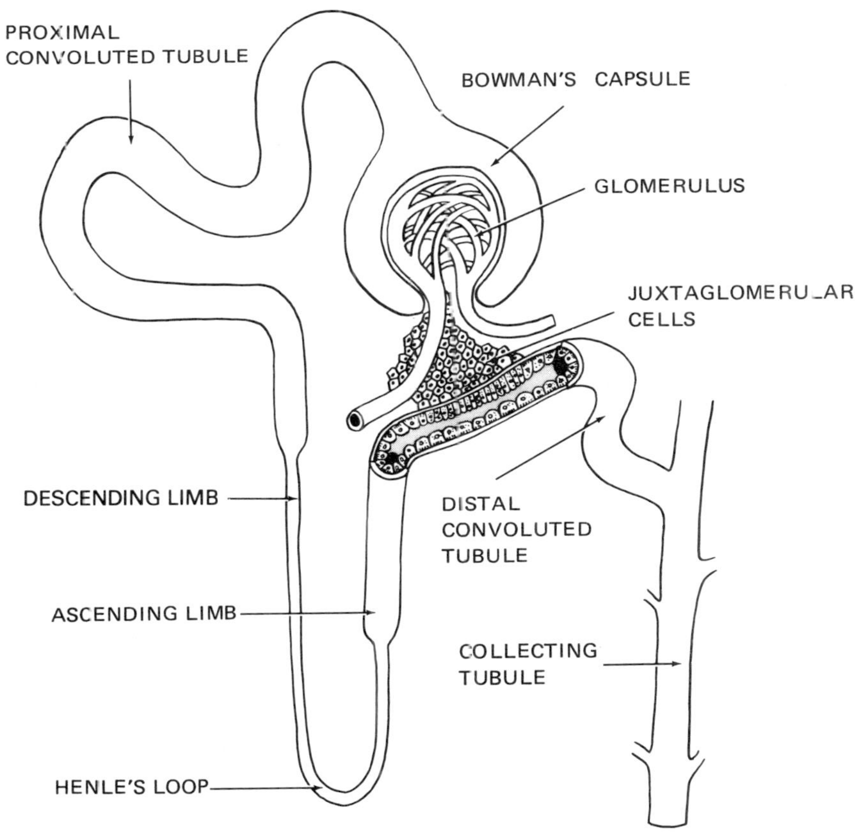


Figure 33

*This is how the system works:*

*Decrease in perfusion pressure ——→ JG cells secrete the enzyme renin ——→ Renin acts on a blood protein to produce angiotensin I and II ——→ Angiotensin II stimulates the adrenal gland to secrete the hormone aldosterone ——→ Aldosterone makes the kidney tubule save more sodium (and water) ——→ Blood volume is expanded, and perfusion pressure in the afferent arteriole is increased.*

*Decreased extracellular concentration of sodium also causes the kidney to release renin, with the saving of sodium as a result.*

## Frame 11

Now test your understanding by outlining the JG system.

1. Stimulus: (increased/decreased) pressure in the afferent arteriole
2. Receptor(s): ____________
3. Location: (proximal/distal) tubule
4. Secrete: ____________
5. Causes formation of: ________ ________
6. Stimulates secretion of: ____________
7. Effect on kidney tubule: (save/excrete) sodium
8. Effect on
   a. extracellular fluid volume: (increased/decreased)
   b. blood pressure: (increased/decreased)
   c. perfusion pressure in afferent arteriole: (increased/decreased)

1. decreased
2. juxtaglomerular cells (JG)
3. distal
4. renin
5. angiotensin I and II
6. aldosterone
7. save
8.
   a. increased
   b. increased
   c. increased

## Frame 12

True or False:

1. ______ The reabsorption of sodium and water by the kidney will reduce blood volume and pressure.

    1. False (More fluid volume in the blood increases the pressure.)

2. ______ Juxtaglomerular cells are located in the glomerulus.

    2. False (They are located in the distal tubule.)

3. ______ Aldosterone influences the kidney to excrete more sodium.

    3. False (Aldosterone causes the kidney to save sodium.)

4. ______ Angiotensin I and II form renin

    4. False (Renin is catalyst for formation of angiotensin.)

5. ______ The juxtaglomerular system is sensitive to changes in perfusion pressure in the afferent arteriole of the kidney.

    5. True

## Frame 13

1. If a patient's systolic blood pressure drops 20 mm Hg, what renal structure(s) will be activated?

    1. Juxtaglomerular cells

2. What enzyme is secreted by the juxtaglomerular cells?

    2. Renin

3. What substance(s) stimulate(s) the adrenal gland to produce aldosterone?

    3. Angiotensin I and II

4. What effect does aldosterone have on the kidney tubules?

    4. Saving of more sodium and water

5. How does this affect the original problem of lowered blood pressure?

    5. Increase in blood volume causes increase in blood pressure

## Frame 14

Summary:

Sodium is the major extracellular ion and is precisely balanced by the kidney tubule.

The proximal tubule reabsorbs much of the filtered sodium; the distal tubule and collecting duct fine-tune the quantity reabsorbed. A number of factors influence this fine-tuning mechanism.

The most important of these are

1. An increase in glomerular filtration rate causes increased sodium reabsorption by the tubules.
2. The juxtaglomerular system: A decrease in perfusion pressure in the afferent arteriole or a decrease in extracellular sodium concentration causes secretion of renin, angiotensin I and II, and aldosterone, which results in increased reabsorption of sodium and water. This increases the blood volume and perfusion pressure.

Some disease processes affecting the kidney tubules cause loss of sodium in the urine.

## CALCIUM AND PHOSPHORUS

### Frame 15

Consider now the renal regulation of calcium (Ca) and phosphorus ($PO_4$).

Calcium is important in blood clotting, transmission of neural impulses and maintaining normal membrane permeability. Phosphate is crucial in formation of ATP, the basic energy source for cells.

There is a continuous two-way movement of calcium and phosphate ions into and out of bone. These two ions do not unite in other tissues, but in bone they combine to form hard crystals which give bone strength. This is caused by a critical ratio of these ions in bone tissue.

Select the statements which correctly describe calcium and phosphorus.

2, 3

1. Calcium and phosphorus circulate in the blood bound together as a compound.
2. Calcium and phosphorus each have different roles in general cellular metabolism.
3. Calcium and phosphorus combine in bone to make hard crystals.
4. Bone strength in weight bearing is unrelated to calcium and phosphorus balance.

### Frame 16

The steady influx of calcium and phosphate ions into bone provides material for continuous remodeling and rebuilding of bone cells.

Calcium can be built into bone only in the presence of phosphorus. The ratio of phosphorus to calcium regulates not only the deposit of calcium, but also the rate of this process.

1. Will a patient with a phosphorus deficiency have less deposit of calcium in his bones?

1. Yes

2. Is it correct to think of bone tissue in the adult as static and unchanging?

2. No

3. What determines the amount of calcium built into bones?

3. Presence of correct amount of phosphorus (along with availability)

## Frame 17

The regulated outflow of calcium from bone enables the body to immediately correct deviations in the blood calcium level. Maintaining serum calcium levels is of highest priority, and calcium will be removed from bone to accomplish it.

True or False:

1. ______ If serum calcium levels are low, problems can result in blood clotting and transmission of nerve impulses.

1. True

2. ______ Once calcium is deposited in bone, it is a permanent part of the structure.

2. False (It can be reabsorbed from bone to replenish blood levels.)

3. ______ Calcium levels in bone and serum are maintained in equilibrium, with serum having priority.

3. True

## Frame 18

Parathyroid hormone (PTH) primarily maintains the serum level of calcium by enhancing calcium and phosphate absorption from the bowel and reabsorption from bone. Under normal conditions, PTH mobilizes calcium from bone at a slow rate, keeping the balance of exit and entry of the ion.

Vitamin D enhances absorption of calcium and phosphate from the bowel and reabsorption from the bone, and it may also enhance calcium and phosphorus combination in bone.

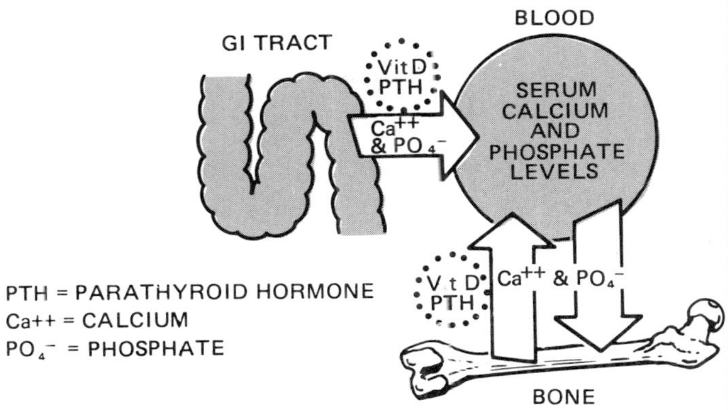


Figure 34

1. If the serum phosphate levels are abnormally low, will calcium be deposited in bone at a normal rate?

2. Does PTH protect the level of calcium in bone or in serum?

1. No (Calcium deposit depends on correct $Ca/PO_4$ ratio.)

2. Serum

## Frame 19

The kidney plays an important role in regulating the blood levels of calcium and phosphorus.

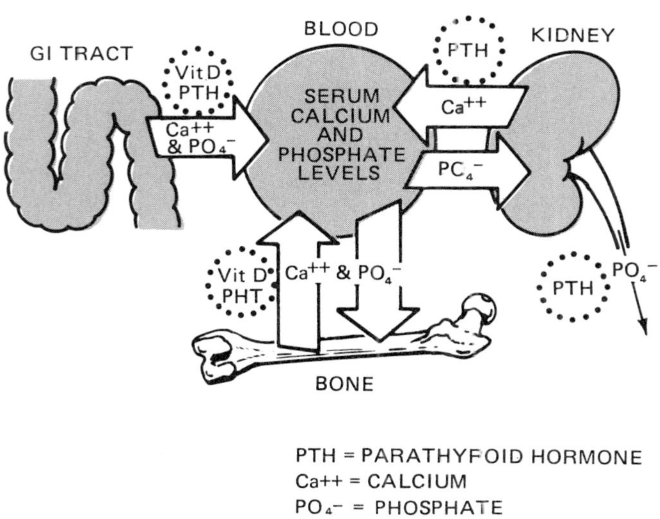


Figure 35

Figures adapted from Neal S. Bricker, ed. *The Sea Within Us*. New York: Science and Medicine Publishing Co, 1975, p. 53.

As the right side of figure 35 demonstrates, PTH influences the kidney to

Reabsorb calcium
Excrete more of the phosphorus.

1. If the serum levels of both calcium and phosphorus were high enough, they could combine and form hard crystals in soft tissue, or renal stones. The kidney prevents this by excreting more (calcium/phosphorus)?

1. phosphorus

2. If the serum calcium level were low, (PTH/Aldosterone) would influence the tubules to reabsorb more calcium?

2. parathyroid hormone (PTH)

3. If serum calcium were high, (more/less) calcium would be reabsorbed by the kidney due to (greater/less) secretion of PTH?

3. less, less

*Panel 2*

***In long-standing renal failure, the following problems related to calcium and phosphorus develop.***

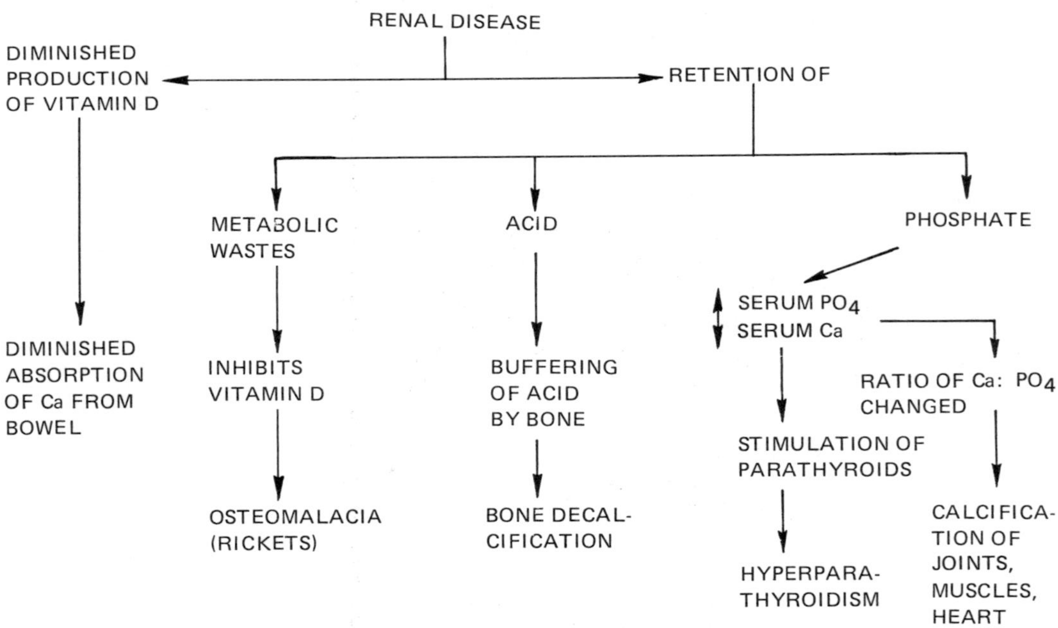


Figure 36

Adapted from Neal S. Bricker, ed. *The Sea Within Us* (N.Y.: Science and Medicine Publ. Co., Inc.) 1975, p. 55.

## Frame 20

Refer to Panel 2 to answer these questions:

1. What three substances are retained by the kidney in renal disease that affect calcium-phosphorus balance?

   1. Metabolic wastes, acids, phosphate

2. How does the retention of $PO_4$ cause the ratio of Ca to $PO_4$ to be changed?
   Serum Ca levels become (high/low).
   Serum $PO_4$ levels become (high/low).

   2. Low
   High

3. Which endocrine glands are stimulated by these blood levels?

   3. Parathyroid

4. What is the outcome of long-term stimulation of the parathyroid gland in renal disease?

   4. Hyperparathyroidism

5. What vitamin is inhibited in renal bone disease?

   5. Vitamin D

## Frame 21

Mr. Evans is in CCU for diagnosis and treatment of possible myocardial infarction. He has had slowly progressing renal failure for the past 7 years. He has some skeletal deformities, old pathologic fractures, and calcium deposits in his soft tissues. He walks with leg braces and crutches.

What are the reason(s) that Mr. Evans has symptoms of bone disease?

a, b, c

a. His kidneys are not efficient in excreting $PO_4$ and saving Ca.

b. Ca is being absorbed from his bones to maintain blood levels.

c. The action of Vitamin D in bone formation is inhibited.

d. None of the above.

## Frame 22

Summary:

Calcium and phosphorus are absorbed from the bowel under the influence of parathyroid hormone and Vitamin D.

Blood calcium and phosphorus levels are in equilibrium with one another and with bone tissue components.

- Calcium and phosphorus combine in bone to form hard crystals. This is regulated by the phosphorus concentration.
- Calcium can be removed from bone to maintain normal serum calcium levels.

Serum levels of calcium and phosphorus affect parathyroid hormone secretion.

Under the influence of parathyroid hormone, the tubules

- Reabsorb calcium ions from the filtrate
- Excrete excess phosphorus.

Failure of the kidney tubules to perform these functions results in bone demineralization and deformities, and soft tissue calcification.

## POTASSIUM

### Frame 23

The last electrolyte to be considered is potassium (K). Potassium is the major intracellular ion and is an important factor in the conduction of nerve impulses in the heart.

Food is a rich source of potassium. After potassium is absorbed from the GI tract, the kidney regulates its serum level. Normally all but 5%–10% of potassium is reabsorbed, and the excess is excreted by the distal tubules in exchange for sodium.

Since the potassium level is dependent on many variable factors, the renal failure patient may have hypo- or hyperkalemia. Here is an example of hypokalemia.

Mrs. White had vomiting and diarrhea along with other symptoms of uremia. She was taking a thiazide diuretic to control edema, which increases excretion of potassium as well as sodium.

1. Choose the routes of loss of K in Mrs. White's case
   a. GI tract
   b. Skin
   c. Kidneys
   d. All of the above

1. a. because of vomiting & diarrhea
   c. due to the effect of the diuretic

2. When potassium loss from the body is in excess of intake, the serum potassium
   a. rises
   b. falls

2. b

### Frame 24

Now consider the potential for hyperkalemia.

Mr. Sidney has acute renal failure following a massive crushing injury. Tissue trauma has released a large amount of potassium from inside the cells. Because Mr. Sidney has loss of renal function and low urine output, the excess potassium ions are not excreted. Hyperkalemia can also become a problem in chronic renal failure, especially if a condition resulting in cell destruction is superimposed.

1. Why is potassium retained in acute renal failure?

2. What effect does trauma to cells have on potassium levels in the blood?

1. If the patient is not producing urine, excess potassium can't be excreted.

2. Raises the blood level because K moves out of cells into the extracellular compartment.

Accumulation of potassium can cause ventricular fibrillation or cardiac arrest.

Serum K $<$ 6.5 mEq/liter is associated with a normal ECG.

Higher levels are associated with cardiac toxicity in varying degrees.

The ECG changes sometimes occur earlier than other symptoms. The general effect of hyperkalemia is interference with the SA node and conduction system. This figure shows the ECG changes that can be expected:

TYPICAL ECG PATTERNS ASSOCIATED WITH ELEVATED SERUM POTASSIUM LEVELS

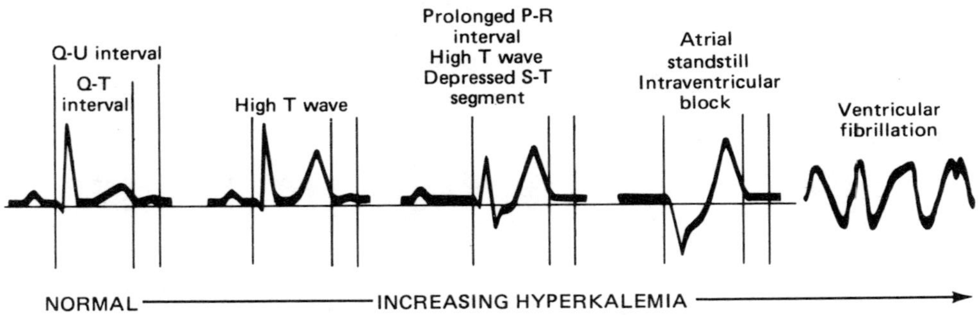


Figure 37

Glenn D. Lubash, "Acute Renal Failure" Hosp Med 1:8, April 1975, p. 15

3. Which of these ECG changes are early effects of hyperkalemia?
   a. No P waves
   b. Prolonged P-R interval
   c. PVCs
   d. Depressed S-T segment
   e. High T wave

3. b, d, e

4. What is the most serious effect of hyperkalemia?

4. Interference with the conduction system of the heart which can cause cardiac arrest

## Frame 25

In chronic renal failure, hyperkalemia is not a serious problem until most of the nephrons are diseased. The intact nephrons' ability to excrete potassium can be increased greatly to compensate for loss of functioning nephrons. If aldosterone and sodium levels are adequate, potassium homeostasis is maintained. However, increased intake of potassium or acidosis can upset this balance.

True or false:

1. ______ The kidney has little reserve capacity to excrete potassium.

1. False

2. ______ Potassium excretion in chronic renal failure depends on the number of functioning nephrons.

2. True

3. ______ Greatly reduced urine output is associated with potassium retention.

3. True

## Frame 26

Summary:

Potassium is released in the GI tract by metabolism of foods.

The kidneys reabsorb most of the potassium and excrete the excess by exchanging potassium ions for sodium and hydrogen ions.

If the nephrons are not able to excrete excess potassium, as in acute renal failure with oliguria or anuria, hyperkalemia results, with cardiac toxicity.

The effect of hyperkalemia on the heart is interference with the conduction of nerve impulses that control heart action.

The nephrons have a great reserve capacity to excrete potassium. In chronic renal failure the intact nephrons can compensate to maintain potassium balance.

A brief review:

## Frame 27

1. Name the hormone that regulates tubular reabsorption of each of these electrolytes:
   a. Calcium
   b. Sodium
   c. Phosphorus
2. For each systemic sign or symptom, name the electrolyte(s) implicated.
   a. Bone demineralization
   b. Cardiac toxicity
   c. Fluid imbalances
   d. Calcification of soft tissue

1.
   a. Parathyroid hormone
   b. Aldosterone
   c. Parathyroid hormone

2.
   a. Calcium and phosphorus
   b. Potassium
   c. Sodium
   d. Calcium and phosphorus

## Frame 28

If a patient has renal failure and has decreased urine output, which of the following problems are likely to develop?

a. Low serum levels of urea, creatinine, and other metabolic wastes
b. Low serum calcium
c. Hyperkalemia
d. High serum phosphorus
e. Dehydration
f. Cardiac arrhythmias

b, c, d, f

# CHAPTER 6

# ASSESSMENT: REABSORPTION AND EXCRETION OF SOLUTES

A number of methods are used to assess the kidney's ability to excrete waste products and to maintain a stable internal environment for the body cells. At the conclusion of this chapter, you will be able to

1. Define clearance
2. Explain the value of creatinine clearance as a test of renal function
3. Differentiate between creatinine clearance and serum creatinine
4. Substantiate the statement: BUN is a less accurate indicator of renal function than creatinine levels.
5. Differentiate between azotemia and uremia
6. Given a list of body systems, list a physical symptom of uremia for each
7. Recognize the systemic effects of electrolyte imbalances frequently seen in renal failure.

## Chapter outline

Clearance
- Definition
- Procedure
- Substances measured
  - Urea
  - Creatinine

Physical signs of uremia
- Skin
- Cardiovascular system
- Nervous system
- Skeletal system

Effects of renal failure on reabsorption and excretion of solutes
- Glucose
- Electrolytes

# PART I
# CLEARANCE

## Frame 1

The effectiveness of the glomerulus as a filter could be measured directly if the amount of urine excreted was the same as the amount of fluid filtered into Bowman's capsule. Direct measurement is not possible since only 1% of filtered water is excreted as urine.

Instead, the *rate* at which substances are removed (cleared) from plasma and excreted in the urine is measured. This is called the *clearance* of a substance. It is expressed as the number of milliliters of plasma cleared of a test substance each minute.

1. The clearance of a substance shows the effectiveness of the (glomerular membrane/distal tubule).
2. Clearance refers to the (filtration/reabsorption) of substances in the blood.
3. Clearance is the amount of (plasma/urine) from which the substance has been removed.

1. glomerular membrane
2. filtration
3. plasma

## Frame 2

Creatinine and urea are two common nitrogenous waste products from protein metabolism that may be measured to determine clearance.

Creatinine is released during metabolism of the body's muscle cells. The amount released is in proportion to the muscle mass of the individual.

A normal serum level is 0–1 mg/100 ml. It is almost completely filtered from the blood and excreted.

Urea is the major end product of protein metabolism. Its greatest source is exogenous (dietary) protein. A normal serum blood urea nitrogen (BUN) level is 10–20 mg/100 ml. Dietary intake of protein as well as catabolism due to infection or injury will raise the BUN level.

Urea, needed for the synthesis of nonessential amino acids, is usually 40%-50% reabsorbed depending on the amount of the urine formed.

| | *Creatinine* | *Urea* |
|---|---|---|
| Source | Muscle activity | Food protein |
| Serum level | 0-1 mg/100 ml | 10-20 mg/100 ml |
| Amount filtered and excreted | Almost 100% | 50%-60% |

True or false:

1. ______ If a man eats a 10-oz steak for dinner, he may later have an increased BUN.
2. ______ More creatinine than urea is reabsorbed by the tubule.

1. True
2. False

## Frame 3

The clearance of creatinine is used most often to assess the level of kidney function. Creatinine is liberated from muscle and excreted in the urine at a fairly constant rate of 1 mg/min. Recall that GFR is approximately 125 ml/min, so the normal rate of clearance of creatinine ($C_{cr}$) is approximately 125 ml of plasma per minute.

Normal values, depending on muscle mass, are
  Males: 100-150 ml/min
  Females: 85-125 ml/min

1. a. Because it is released, filtered, and excreted at a fairly constant rate of 1 mg/min, (urea/creatinine) is the substance used to determine glomerular filtration rate.
   b. Since glomerular filtration rate is computed to be 125 ml/min, it can be said that $C_{cr}$ (does/does not) reflect true GFR.
   c. A large muscular person would normally have (higher/lower) creatinine levels than a petite person.
2. Which is the less accurate indicator of renal function, BUN or creatinine?
3. What does the abbreviation $C_{cr}$ signify?

1. a. creatinine
   b. does
   c. higher
2. BUN
3. Clearance of creatinine

## Frame 4

Between the ages of 40 and 80 the glomerular filtration rate, or clearance, drops so that by age 80 a normal $C_{cr}$ might be 60–65 ml/min.

1. The process of aging (decreases/increases) GFR and clearance.
2. This implies that the kidney (does/does not) have the ability to renew itself.
3. Ms. Allen, who is 72, has a $C_{cr}$ of 72 ml/min. This indicates a (normal/abnormal) level of function for her kidneys.

1. decreases
2. does not
3. normal

## Frame 5

Initially, a patient's $C_{cr}$ is determined to provide a baseline assessment of kidney function. Then the serum creatinine ($S_{cr}$) levels are routinely used to monitor kidney function, as this is a much simpler procedure. Significant changes in the $S_{cr}$ would indicate the need to again determine $C_{cr}$.

True or false:

1. ______ A rapid rise in $S_{cr}$ indicates a rapid progression of kidney disease.
2. ______ $S_{cr}$ is used as a routine monitoring test to determine rate and direction of changes in renal function.
3. ______ Creatinine clearance is a measurement of *rate* at which creatinine is removed from the plasma and excreted.
4. ______ Serum creatinine is a measurement of the *amount* of creatinine in the plasma.
5. ______ If a patient has a creatinine clearance of 1 mg/100 ml, the lab report is erroneous.

1. True
2. True
3. True
4. True
5. True ($C_{cr}$ measures *rate* of clearance and is reported in the unit milliliters per minute.)

## Frame 6

Identify reasons why it can be said that serum creatinine is a more specific and sensitive indicator of renal function than BUN. (Hint: see Frames 2 and 3.)

BUN is influenced by more variables: that is, dietary intake of protein, increased protein catabolism (infection, injury), reabsorption. Creatinine is released, filtered, and excreted at a fairly constant rate.

## Frame 7

In order to measure creatinine clearance, it is necessary to use the entire volume of urine excreted during a specific time period. The procedure for collecting the specimens for a clearance is as follows:

Empty bladder and discard this urine. Note this time as the beginning of the collection.

Save all urine for next 24 hours (or number of hours specified).

Void exactly 24 hours later (or at a specified time). Save this urine and send the total specimen to the laboratory.

A blood sample to measure serum creatinine is drawn during the 24-hour time period.

In the following two cases choose the course of action you should take:

1. The patient is unable to void at 24 hours. The previous voiding was at 18 hours.
   a. Send specimen as a 24-hour collection.
   b. Send specimen as an 18-hour collection.

1. b (The exact number of hours and minutes is a very important component in figuring an accurate clearance. It is equally important to have all the urine.)

2. The patient is incontinent of a large amount of urine.
   a. Restart the urine collection.
   b. Deduct an estimated amount of urine from the collection.
   c. Continue the collection as if it didn't happen.

2. a

## Frame 8

The formula to determine clearance is

$$C = \frac{\text{Urine concentration (mg/100 ml)} \times \text{Urine flow (ml/min)}}{\text{Serum concentration (mg/100 ml)}}$$

Mrs. Rice's urine creatinine concentration in the 24-hour specimen was 30 mg.

$$C = \frac{30 \times \text{Urine flow}}{\text{Serum concentration}}$$

Her urine volume was 1500 ml in 24 hours. To calculate urine flow, divide the volume by the number of minutes (24 hours = 1440 minutes).

$$C = \frac{30 \times \frac{1500}{1440}}{\text{Serum concentration}}$$

The serum concentration was 6.5 mg/100 ml, so

$$C = \frac{30 \times \frac{1500}{1440}}{6.5} = 4.8 \text{ ml/min}$$

1. Is Mrs. Rice in renal failure? (Hint: see Frame 3.)
2. Can you define clearance?

1. Yes
2. The rate at which a volume of plasma is cleared of a substance

3. Find Mr. Johnson's creatinine clearance.

   Urine creatinine = 50 mg
   Urine volume = 2 liters/24 hours (remember to convert to milliliters and minutes)
   Serum creatinine = 2 mg

3. 34.5 ml/min

$$\frac{50 \times \frac{2000\text{ ml}}{1440\text{ min}}}{2} =$$

$$\frac{50 \times 1.38}{2} = \frac{69}{2} = 34.5\text{ ml/min}$$

**Frame 9**

1. Mr. Jamison has had a creatinine clearance test ordered to evaluate his renal function. On the basis of your calculations in the last frame, list what information is needed for this test.

   a.

   b.

   c.

   d.

   a. Urine volume
   b. Time
   c. Serum creatinine
   d. Urine creatinine

2. Place a check before the components that depend on accurate nursing measures.

   Urine volume, time

Computing clearance is usually done by the laboratory personnel, and the patient's height and weight are also considered in correcting the computation. Now that you have done the math, you can understand the importance of the accuracy of nursing procedures related to these tests.

## Frame 10

Summary:

Clearance is the rate at which dissolved substances are removed (cleared) from the plasma and excreted in the urine, expressed in milliliters per minute.

The test is conducted by analyzing a 24-hour urine specimen for concentration of the substance, and comparing this with the serum level of the substance.

Creatinine is released during muscle metabolism and is completely filtered and excreted by the normal kidney. It is not influenced by other factors, and is therefore an accurate indicator of renal clearance.

Normal values are
Males: 100–150 ml/min
Females: 85–125 ml/min
Both by age 80: 60–65 ml/min

The serum creatinine is used on a routine basis to monitor kidney function.

Normal: 0–1 mg/100 ml

The BUN measures the amount of urea in the serum. Urea is not completely excreted by the normal kidney and is influenced by dietary intake of protein, and by infection and injury. Thus it is a less accurate indicator of renal function.

Normal: 10–20 mg/100 ml

# PART II PHYSICAL SIGNS OF UREMIA

Due to decreased filtration and excretion in renal failure, urea, creatinine, uric acid, and other substances accumulate and cause toxic effects on most body systems.

## Frame 11

*Azotemia* refers to a high concentration of nitrogenous wastes in the blood.

Would an azotemic patient have high or low blood levels of urea, uric acid, and creatinine? — High

*Uremia* refers to the syndrome seen in end-stage renal conditions. The uremic syndrome is caused by the retention of the products of nitrogen metabolism (azotemia) and the changes that occur in water, electrolyte, and acid-base balances.

Match each term to its definition:

a. Azotemia  b. Uremia

1. ______ The presence of nitrogenous waste products in the blood — 1. a
2. ______ The clinical manifestations of renal failure — 2. b

## Frame 12

Mrs. Rice has a BUN of 126 mg/100 ml and a creatinine of 9.18 mg/100 ml.

1. Is Mrs. Rice azotemic or uremic? — 1. Azotemic
2. If Mrs. Rice also had uremia, physical symptoms would occur due to: — 2. a, b, c, d
   a. Azotemia
   b. Electrolyte imbalance
   c. Fluid balance disturbance
   d. Acid-base imbalance
   e. None of the above

## SKIN

### Frame 13

The skin attempts to excrete some of the waste products accumulated due to renal failure, and as this occurs, the skin may show color and texture changes:

The patient's skin may be a yellow tan due to the presence of urochrome, a pigment that gives urine its normal color.

The patient may have a white powdery substance on the skin. This is from the formation of urate crystals and is referred to as "uremic frost." Uremic frost is seldom seen, as dialysis is usually begun before the patient reaches this terminal state.

1. In patients with renal failure the skin becomes __________________ in color due to retention of ____________.

1. yellow tan
   urochrome

2. Uremic frost is an excretion of ____________ crystals by the skin which occurs (early/late) in the disease.

2. urate, late

### Frame 14

Patients in renal failure complain of intense itching (pruritus). The cause is not fully understood but perhaps the retained toxins irritate the nerve fibers in the skin. Calcium imbalances are also involved.

Choose the common things to look for in the patient with pruritus:

a. Numerous scratch marks
b. Continuous scratching
c. Complaints of itching
d. Skin that is smooth and waxlike
e. Skin that seems rough and dry

a, b, c, e

## CARDIOVASCULAR SYSTEM

### Frame 15

The metabolic imbalances seem to interfere with the normal adhesiveness of platelets. The number of platelets is normal, but bleeding time is increased. This clotting defect may be one reason renal failure patients do not generally have problems with phlebitis and pulmonary emboli.

Which of these cardiovascular signs or symptoms might you observe in a renal failure patient?

a. Decreased number of platelets
b. Bruises
c. Difficulty stopping the bleeding after a venipuncture

b, c (These are all signs of increased bleeding time. The number of platelets is usually normal.)

### Frame 16

It is common for patients with renal failure to have anemia. This is due in part to a decreased production of erythropoietin, a hormone secreted by the kidneys. This hormone stimulates bone marrow to produce red blood cells. The patients' other metabolic imbalances also decrease the normal life span of mature red blood cells. Often their hemoglobin ranges 6–10 g/100 ml.

Mark these statements true or false:

1. ______ A patient in renal failure would have a hemoglobin around 8 g/100 ml.
2. ______ Such a patient would be pale and easily fatigued.

1. True
2. True

## Frame 17

The toxic metabolic imbalances associated with renal failure are also thought to be involved in uremic pericarditis. (The pericardium is the serous membrane surrounding the heart.) This is different from bacterial pericarditis as there is usually no infection. The toxins cause inflammation and fibrous changes in the pericardium. There may be no signs or symptoms or there may be a friction rub, low grade fever, hypotension or chest pain or any combination.

Mrs. Rice is being observed for pericarditis because her blood pressure drops during dialysis and doesn't respond to fluid replacement. Of the following, choose the signs or symptoms that pertain to pericarditis.

a. Temperature of $99^4$–$99^8$ for the last 3 days
b. Hypertension
c. A pericardial friction rub
d. Pain in the chest, increased with respiration

a, c, d

## NERVOUS SYSTEM

### Frame 18

The toxic effects on the *central* nervous system are quite variable in different patients. About the earliest symptom is an impaired ability to concentrate. Some patients are agitated and some disoriented, while others are lethargic or even comatose.

List the parameters you would observe to assess the neurologic status of a patient in renal failure.

Levels of consciousness: alert, restless, lethargic, comatose?

Orientation: to time, place, person, self?

Other symptoms that may be pertinent are: Response: to simple commands, to painful stimuli? Are they purposeful, nonpurposeful, or is there no response?

### Frame 19

The patient may complain of numbness and tingling or burning in the extremities and painful walking. This is due to toxic effects on the *peripheral* nervous system. Nerve conduction velocity tests show a slowed response.

True or false:

1. ______ The patient should be observed for changes in gait.
2. ______ If nerve impulses are traveling more slowly than normal, the patient's reflexes will be slower.

1. True
2. True

## SKELETAL SYSTEM

### Frame 20

Uric acid is an end-product of purine metabolism (a nitrogen compound found in meats, beans, peas, coffee, spices, and other foods). Uric acid is elevated in gout and in renal failure. Symptoms attributed to gout are inflammed, swollen, and painful joints, especially of the great toe.

Mark these statements true or false:

1. _____ A patient in renal failure with an elevated uric acid and painful or swollen joints may have gout.

2. _____ A patient with gout has renal failure.

1. True

2. False

# PART III REABSORPTION AND EXCRETION OF GLUCOSE AND ELECTROLYTES

In Chapter 5 you learned that threshold substances such as glucose are reabsorbed or excreted in response to the body's needs.

## Frame 21

In renal failure, the kidney is unable to excrete excess substances.

1. In renal failure will the urine level of glucose reflect the true serum level?
2. Why would a Clinitest for glycosuria be inaccurate for a diabetic in renal failure?

Answers:

1. No
2. The patient may have a high serum glucose and be able to excrete only a trace amount of sugar in the urine.

## Frame 22

In acute renal failure, the kidney loses its normal salt conserving mechanisms. (Normal serum Na = 135–145 mEq/L).

1. Mr. Jamison's *serum* sodium would be (increased/decreased) if he had this problem.
2. This indicates damage to the (glomerulus/tubule).
3. What hormone is ineffective at this time?

Answers:

1. decreased (Sodium is not reabsorbed.)
2. tubule
3. Aldosterone

## Frame 23

The patient in chronic failure will not be able to conserve sodium in certain diseases that affect the tubule such as pyelonephritis.

1. Select the correct words:
   a. Chronic problems with sodium loss indicate (glomerular/tubular) damage.
   b. Since sodium losses lead to hypovolemia, low serum sodium (will/will not) contribute to poor perfusion of the kidney.

Answers:

1.
   a. tubular
   b. will (↓ Na → ↓ blood volume → ↓ kidney perfusion)

2. What effect does decreased perfusion have on kidney function?

2. It decreases glomerular filtration, thus contributing to progression of renal failure.

## Frame 24

Excretion of excess Magnesium (Mg) is another normal kidney function that is lost in renal failure. Mg is only present in small amounts (normal serum = 1.5–2.5 mEq/liter) but it is necessary for cell function. Five to ten times the normal level can cause CNS depression. It is important to know if the patient has been using preparations high in magnesium such as Mylanta, milk of magnesia or Maalox.

Mr. Reynolds is having an episode of renal failure following upper gastrointestinal hemorrhage and shock. He has taken Maalox for his gastric ulcers for years and is asking to have this medication continued.

1. Why might Maalox cause a problem for Mr. Reynolds?

1. In renal failure the kidney tubules can't excrete excess magnesium.

2. What is the result of high blood levels of magnesium?

2. CNS depression

## Frame 25

Bone disease associated with renal failure may be characterized by softening and demineralizing of the bones. Patients may complain of bone pain. Fractures may easily occur.

1. Choose the correct ions in parentheses to complete this statement: Renal bone disease is a result of imbalances of (Na/Cl/Ca/$PO_4$). (If you need to review this, see Chapter 5, Frames 15–22.)

1. Ca, $PO_4$

2. What hormone would probably be elevated due to this imbalance?
3. What vitamin has been interfered with?
4. What normal kidney functions are lost?
   a. (Excretion/Reabsorption) of calcium
   b. (Excretion/Reabsorption) of phosphorus
5. In renal failure the serum phosphorus (increases/decreases) and the serum calcium (increases/decreases).

2. PTH
3. Vitamin D
4.
   a. Reabsorption
   b. Excretion
5. increases
   decreases

**Frame 26**

The potassium level becomes one of the most important problems in acute renal failure but is less of a problem in chronic failure until most nephrons are damaged. (Normal serum K = 3.5–5.5 mEq/L.)

1. Why is potassium retained in renal failure?
2. Choose the signs or symptoms of hyperkalemia:
   a. Bradycardia
   b. Spiked T-waves and wide QRS interval
   c. Hypertension
3. What is the most serious effect of hyperkalemia?

1. The kidneys can no longer excrete the excess potassium.
2. a, b
3. Ventricular fibrillation or cardiac arrest

**Frame 27**

Some other factors can aggravate hyperkalemia in patients with renal failure. These are

Increased dietary intake of food high in potassium, such as dried fruits and nuts

Blood transfusions followed by hemolysis of red blood cells, which liberates the intracellular potassium

Use of salt substitutes that are potassium salts

Infection

Uncontrolled acidosis, because the kidney excretes hydrogen ions and keeps $K^+$.

*Hypokalemia* may also be seen in patients with renal failure when there are

Increased losses of $K^+$ due to vomiting and diarrhea, or diuretics that influence the kidney to excrete $K^+$.

Decreased intake in nausea or anorexia.

Hypokalemia may cause fatigue, muscle weakness and cardiac dysrhythmias.

Match each situation with its probable effect in a renal failure patient.

a. Hyperkalemia　　b. Hypokalemia

| | | | Answer |
|---|---|---|---|
| 1. | ______ | High intake of dried fruits | 1. a |
| 2. | ______ | Vomiting and diarrhea | 2. b |
| 3. | ______ | Blood transfusion with hemolysis | 3. a |
| 4. | ______ | Infection | 4. a |
| 5. | ______ | Loss of appetite with poor food intake | 5. b |
| 6. | ______ | Diabetic acidosis | 6. a |
| 7. | ______ | Use of potassium-based salt substitutes | 7. a |

## Frame 28

Here is a list of signs and symptoms seen in renal failure:

a. Calcium deposits under the skin
b. Impaired concentration
c. Low grade fever
d. ECG changes
e. Uremic frost
f. Purpura
g. Lethargy
h. Decreased nerve conduction velocity
i. Yellow tan color or urochrome
j. Bruises
k. Fractures
l. Pericardial friction rub
m. Bone pain
n. Pruritus
o. Dysrhythmias

1. Which symptoms are due to the skin's excretory activity?
2. Which are caused by decreased adhesiveness of platelets and a clotting defect?
3. Which reflect central and peripheral nerve disturbances?
4. Which are signs of the bone disease common in renal patients?
5. Which are due to potassium imbalances?
6. Which are characteristic of pericarditis?

1. e, i, n
2. f, j
3. b, g, h
4. a, k, m
5. d, o
6. c, l

## Frame 29

Summary:

Azotemia is increased serum concentration of nitrogenous wastes such as urea, uric acid, and creatinine.

Uremia is the syndrome caused by azotemia and imbalances of water, electrolytes, and buffers, seen in late stages of chronic renal failure.

Skin: yellowish color, pruritus, uremic frost present in late stage
CNS: impaired concentration, restlessness, disorientation, lethargy, coma
Peripheral neuropathy
Cardiovascular: defect in platelet function with prolonged bleeding time, uremic pericarditis, dysrhythmias due to potassium imbalances
Bone: demineralization, softening, gout due to increased uric acid

Electrolyte imbalances frequently seen in renal failure are

1. Increased serum potassium, magnesium, phosphorus
2. Decreased serum calcium, sodium, and sometimes potassium

# CHAPTER 7

## BODY FLUID BALANCE

Water is the greatest single component of the body, representing about 60% of the total body weight of an adult. Intake of water is variable and capricious. Water loss is also variable, depending on the environment. You will now look at the kidney's role in precisely regulating this crucial element. At the end of this chapter, you will be able to

1. Explain the effect of osmosis on body water dynamics
2. Define osmolality
3. Describe the effects of change in sodium concentration on extracellular fluid volume
4. Explain the kidney tubule's method of separating water and electrolytes
5. List factors that influence secretion of ADH
6. State the effect of ADH on tubular reabsorption of water
7. Relate tubular reabsorption of water to urine osmolality and volume
8. Recognize symptoms of impairment of concentration mechanisms
9. Recognize symptoms of impairment of dilution mechanisms.

### Chapter outline

# PART I
# REVIEW OF FUNDAMENTAL CONCEPTS

Before studying the kidney's role in regulating body water, you may need to review some basic principles.

## Body Fluid Compartments

### Frame 1

The fluid compartments of the body are important because significant shifts can take place between them.

The *intra*cellular compartment means all of the water within the cells.

Where is the intracellular fluid in the cell in this figure?

Between the nucleus and cell membrane

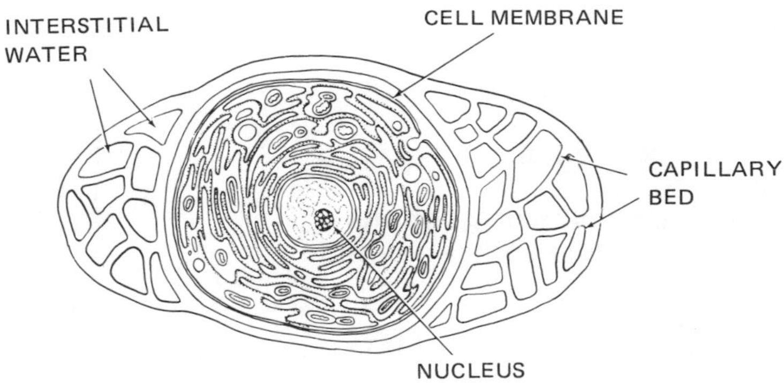


Figure 38

The *extra*cellular compartment is all of the body water outside of the cells. This includes:

The blood plasma
The interstitial fluid, around the outside of cells.

Because of osmosis, fluid moves back and forth between the compartments.

1. If the blood has higher osmotic pressure (therefore, more dissolved particles) than the interstitial fluid, which way will fluid move?

1. From interstitial fluid to blood

2. If the interstitial fluid is more concentrated than the blood which way will fluid move?

2. From blood to interstitial fluid

## Chemical and Osmotic Activity of Solutions

### Frame 2

Each of the water compartments of the body contains a differing concentration and composition of electrolytes. The *physical and chemical* activity of electrolytes (as in diffusion) depends on the *number of electric charges* per unit of volume, expressed as equivalents or milliequivalents per liter (mEq).

1. In the solution in this figure, how many electric charges are present?

1. 20

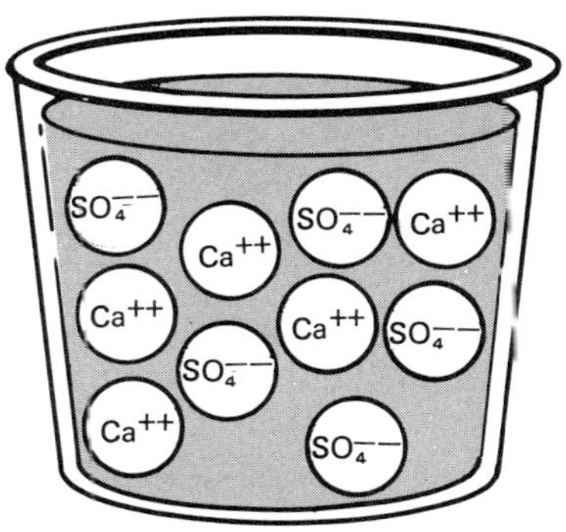


Figure 39

2. How would the number of electric charges in the solution be expressed?

2. 20 milliequivalents (mEq)

## Frame 3

The *osmotic* activity of a solution depends on the *number of particles* dissolved in solution (the charges they carry have no relationship to osmotic activity). They are expressed as milli-osmols (mOsm).

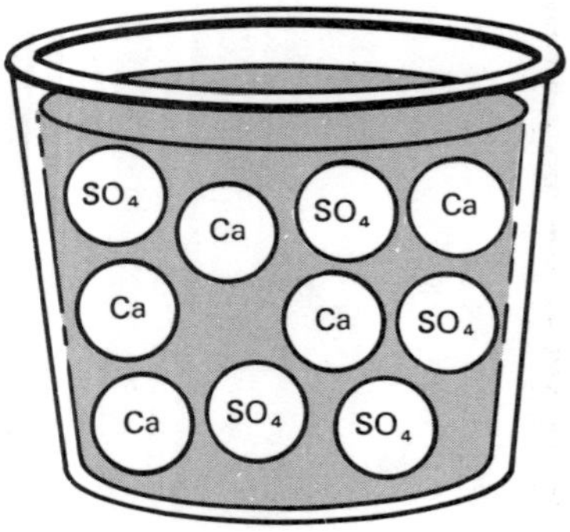


Figure 40

1. How many particles are present in this figure?
2. How would the osmotic activity of this solution be expressed?

1. 10

2. 10 milliosmols

The milliosmol measures the amount of work dissolved particles can do in drawing fluid through a semipermeable membrane, or the osmotic pressure of the solution.

Which of the following solutions has the highest osmotic pressure?

a. 20 mOsm
b. 50 mOsm
c. 70 mEq

b (Milliequivalents measure chemical activity or the number of electric bonds available.)

### Osmotic Activity in Body Fluid Compartments

## Frame 4

When looking at the body's fluid balance, terms are needed to express the osmotic activity of the fluid in each compartment.

An *isotonic* solution has the same number of dissolved particles and the same osmotic pressure as another solution.

1. If plasma, interstitial fluid, and intracellular fluid are all isotonic, which way will fluid move between them?

1. Fluid will not move between them, as osmotic pressure is equal.

2. a. An IV solution is considered isotonic if it has the same ____________ pressure as body fluid.
   b. This is dependent on the ____________ of dissolved particles.

2.
a. osmotic
b. number

## Frame 5

If one body fluid compartment has more dissolved particles than another, the fluid is called *hypertonic,* or concentrated.

1. A hypertonic solution has (higher/lower) osmotic pressure.

1. higher

2. Mr. Williams was given an IV infusion of albumin. This would (increase/decrease) the osmotic pressure of the blood.

2. increase (Albumin is a blood protein. More osmotic particles are being added.)

3. If Mr. William's plasma were hypertonic as compared to interstitial fluid, fluid would move from (interstitial space to blood/blood to interstitial space).

3. interstitial space to blood

4. Mrs. Harris is dehydrated following severe, untreated vomiting and diarrhea. Because of loss of body water, her blood would have (more/less) dissolved particles per unit volume. Her plasma is now (isotonic/hypertonic) compared to its concentration before her illness.

4. more
hypertonic

## Frame 6

A solution having fewer dissolved particles is called *hypotonic,* or dilute.

1. Fewer dissolved particles means (higher/lower) osmotic pressure.

1. lower

2. Mrs. Elmore has acute glomerulonephritis and has 4+ proteinuria, with a serum albumin of 2.0 (normal = 3.2 - 5.6). Her plasma would be (hypo/hyper) tonic compared to interstitial fluid, and fluid would move from the __________ to the __________ compartment.

2. hypotonic
blood, interstitial

## Frame 7

This figure shows the three body fluid compartments:

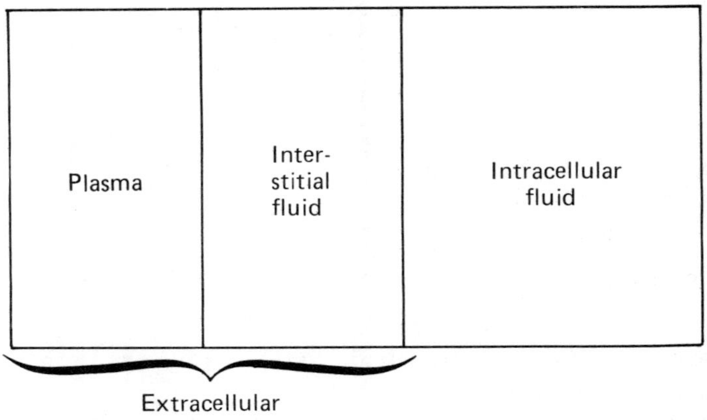


Figure 41

Plasma and interstitial fluid are commonly considered together as the extracellular fluid.

Plasma is the fluid component of circulating blood. It is made up of 92% water, 6%-8% protein, and variable amounts of carbohydrates, lipids, electrolytes, and metabolic waste products. Sometimes the plasma is called the vascular compartment.

The interstitial fluid is found in all parts of the body, between and in body cavities. The cells of the body live in it. Nutrient materials and oxygen pass through the walls of the capillaries and through tissue fluid to reach cells. So interstitial fluid is the "middleman" for exchanges between blood and cells. The composition of tissue fluid is nearly identical to plasma, except that it has less protein than plasma and more chloride.

Fill in the blanks to complete these statements:

1. The fluid compartments of the body are _________, _________, and _________.

2. Two compartments comprise the extracellular fluid, these are __________ and __________.

3. Components that give plasma its osmotic pressure are __________, __________, __________, __________, and __________ __________. (Hint: What are the dissolved particles?)

Answers:

1. plasma (or vascular), interstitial, intracellular
2. plasma interstitial
3. protein, electrolytes, lipids, carbohydrates, metabolic wastes

## Frame 8

Match each term with a related idea. If you have problems with any of these, review the frame indicated.

1. _______Milliequivalents (Frame 2)
2. _______Hypertonic solution (Frame 5)
3. _______Milliosmols (Frame 3)
4. _______Extracellular fluid compartment (Frame 7)
5. _______Hypotonic solution (Frame 6)
6. _______Vascular fluid compartment (Frame 7)
7. _______Isotonic (Frame 4)

a. Low osmotic pressure
b. Blood plasma
c. Movement of water from areas of high to low concentration of particles
d. Chemical activity relative to the number of electric charges
e. High osmotic pressure
f. Osmotic activity relative to the total number of particles present
g. Same number of particles in each of two solutions
h. Interstitial fluid and plasma
i. Measurement of the weight of dissolved particles

Answers:

1. d
2. e
3. f
4. h
5. a
6. b
7. g

# PART II
# KIDNEY REGULATION OF WATER

## Frame 9

As discussed earlier, there is a wide variability in the amount of fluid a person takes in and loses each day. Therefore, the kidney's ability to save and excrete water through concentrating and diluting urine is vital to the dynamic equilibrium of body fluid.

Water is the least restricted and least confined substance in the body. It continually flows through cell membranes from one body fluid compartment to another. But its movement is governed by osmosis. In imbalanced states, water will flow between the cell and extracellular fluid according to osmotic gradients, even if the shift jeopardizes life.

Respond true or false to the following statements:

1. ______ Most cell membranes are not permeable to water.
2. ______ Water must follow osmotic gradients between the body fluid compartments until the extracellular and intracellular fluid concentrations are balanced.
3. ______ The osmotic pressure in the extracellular compartment determines the water content of the cells.

1. False
2. True
3. True

## Frame 10

Outside the cells the particles causing osmotic pressure are mainly sodium, chloride, bicarbonate, and glucose.

Inside the cells, there is a comparable number of osmotically active particles—potassium, magnesium, sulfate, and phosphate.

Much of the cell's energy is devoted to maintaining this separation of osmotically active particles in extracellular and intracellular compartments.

The total number of osmotically active particles per liter of solution is called *osmolality.*

1. Complete the following statement
   If extra particles of sodium are added to the extracellular fluid (ECF), the osmolality will be (increased/decreased) and water will shift (into/out of) the cells.

1. increased
   out of

Mr. Richards was given hypertonic sodium bicarbonate (IV) in large amounts during treatment for cardiac arrest. The resuscitation was successful, but several hours later he had symptoms of water intoxication with increased CVP, pulmonary edema, and convulsions.

2. Where did the extra load of water in the vascular and interstitial spaces come from?
   a. From increased oral intake
   b. From the *intra*cellular space
   c. Neither of the above

2. b

3. What caused this massive redistribution of body water?
   a. The sodium bicarbonate increased osmotic pressure in the blood, drawing fluid in.
   b. This is a side effect of pressure during cardiac massage.
   c. Neither of the above.

3. a

*Panel 1*

*You have seen that water is usually locked into an osmotic relationship with electrolytes. In order to regulate the osmolality of ECF, water must be isolated from the electrolytes and regulated as a separate entity.*

*As you read trace the steps involved in the kidney's method of water control shown in the figure.*

1. *Delivery: Filtrate is delivered to the Loop of Henle after about two thirds of the water has been reabsorbed by osmosis from the proximal tubule.*
2. *Separation: Chloride ($Cl^-$) is pumped out of the ascending limb of Henle's loop, and sodium ($Na^+$) follows along the electric gradient created. This part of the tubule is watertight, so water cannot follow osmotic gradients.*

THE THREE BASIC FACTORS IN RENAL WATER CONTROL

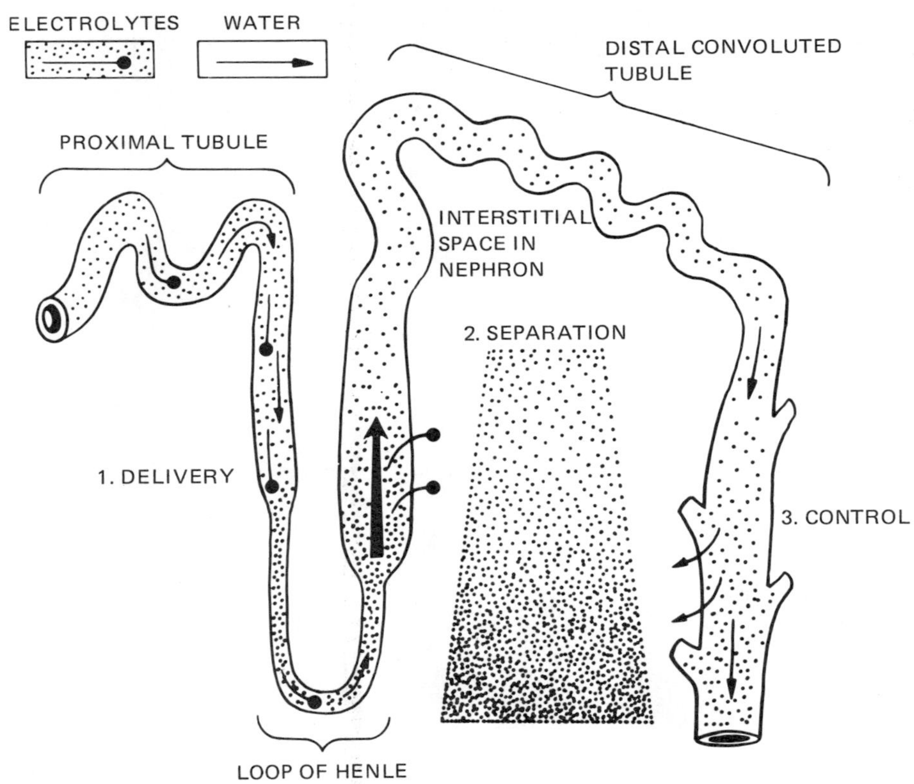


Figure 42

Neal S. Bricker, ed. *The Sea Within Us* (N.Y.: Science and Medicine Publ. Co., Inc.) 1975, p. 97.

3. *Control*

   *The water continues through the distal tubule, which is also watertight, and is excreted as urine. This mechanism will excrete large volumes of excess water.*

   *If water needs to be saved, antidiuretic hormone (ADH) is secreted by the posterior pituitary gland. ADH relaxes the watertightness of the distal tubule, allowing a precise amount of water to be reabsorbed by osmosis. The water that is reabsorbed returns to the peritubular capillaries to replenish blood volume. A much smaller amount of urine is then excreted.*

## Frame 11

1. What physical law governs the movement of water in the body?
2. What hormone affects the distal tubule's permeability to water?

True or false:

3. _______ The reason water is separated from electrolytes in the kidney is to remove it from the control of osmosis.
4. _______ If water is made electrolyte-free in the kidney tubule, it can be saved or excreted according to the body's water needs.

Answers:

1. Osmosis
2. ADH
3. True
4. True

## Frame 12

Match each function with the segment of nephron responsible: (Hint: See Panel 1.)

| | Function | | Segment |
|---|---|---|---|
| 1. | _____ Removal of chloride and sodium from filtrate | a. | Glomerulus |
| 2. | _____ Reabsorption of two thirds of the water | b. | Proximal tubule |
| 3. | _____ Varying amount of water released for osmotic movement | c. | Loop of Henle |
| 4. | _____ Formation of 180 liters filtrate per day | d. | Distal tubule |

Answers:

1. c
2. b
3. d
4. a

## Frame 13

Summary:

Water moves freely between the body fluid compartments according to the law of osmosis.

Osmotic gradients (or pressure) are caused by the number of osmotically active particles per liter of solution. This is called the osmolality and expressed as milliosmols per kilogram (mOsm/Kg).

Intracellular particles are potassium, magnesium, sulfate, and phosphate.

Extracellular particles are sodium, chloride, bicarbonate, and glucose.

The kidney separates water from the electrolytes, thereby freeing it from gradients, and regulates it separately.

1. Delivery: Filtrate is delivered to the Loop of Henle with two thirds of the water already reabsorbed in the proximal tubule.
2. Separation: Chloride is pumped out of the Loop of Henle, sodium follows the electric diffusion gradient out of the tubule, and water is kept in the tubule because the walls are impermeable to water.
3. Control: The distal tubule's wall becomes more permeable to water under the influence of ADH, thus allowing some water to be reabsorbed by osmosis.

# PART III ANTIDIURETIC HORMONE

## Frame 14

Now look at the system that regulates antidiuretic hormone secretion and water balance.

1. Recall the effects of ingesting a large amount of water
   1. The plasma osmolality is (increased/decreased).
   2. The interstitial fluid will then (gain/lose) water, making its osmolality (higher/lower).

Specialized groups of nerve cells called osmoreceptors, which are located in the brain near the hypothalamus, sense this change in osmolality of extracellular fluid. They *inhibit* the secretion of ADH and its release by the pituitary gland.

As a result of curtailed ADH release, the distal tubule remains relatively watertight, not much water is reabsorbed, and a large amount of water is excreted.

The same stimuli that act on osmoreceptors also affect the thirst center in the brain, suppressing thirst and preventing more intake.

3. The stimulus for the level of ADH secretion is the ________ of extracellular fluid.
4. This change is sensed by the ________ in the ________.
5. *Less* ADH secretion causes the ________ tubule to become ________ permeable to water.
6. *Decreasing* ADH secretion results in excretion of (more/less) water.

1. decreased (More water with fewer particles per unit volume)
2. gain lower
3. osmolality
4. osmoreceptors brain (hypothalamus)
5. distal, less
6. more

## Frame 15

1. If the kidneys are excreting more water there will be (more/fewer) dissolved particles in each volume of urine.
2. Urine of low osmolality is (concentrated/dilute).
3. Inhibition of ADH secretion results in a (large/small) volume of urine with (high/low) osmolality.

1. fewer
2. dilute
3. large
   low

## Frame 16

Fill in the blanks describing what happens when a patient becomes dehydrated, or has low blood volume:

1. The plasma osmolality is ____________.
2. Water shifts from the ____________ to the ____________ compartment.

The osmoreceptors detect this interstitial fluid change and *stimulate* the secretion of ADH.

3. ADH (increases/decreases) the distal tubule's permeability to water.
4. In the presence of ADH, the tubules will (excrete/save) more water, because osmosis draws the water (into/out of) the tubule.
5. The water reabsorbed from the tubule is returned via (osmosis/diffusion) to the peritubular capillary, replenishing (blood volume/intracellular volume).

1. increased
2. interstitial
   plasma
3. increases
4. save
   out of
5. osmosis
   blood volume

## Frame 17

1. If water is reabsorbed by the kidney in response to dehydration, the urine excreted will have (more/fewer) particles dissolved in each unit volume.
2. Urine of high osmolality is (dilute/concentrated).
3. ADH secretion results in a (large/small) volume of urine with (high/low) osmolality.

1. more
2. concentrated
3. small
   high

## Frame 18

Fill in the chart describing each step involved in correcting the fluid imbalance. Refer to Frame 20 if you need to.

| | Dehydration | Large fluid load |
|---|---|---|
| 1. ECF osmolality | | |
| 2. Sensed by | | |
| 3. ADH secretion | | |
| 4. Kidney tubules' permeability to water | | |
| 5. Amount of water returned to blood | | |
| 6. Amount of urine | | |
| 7. Urine osmolality | | |

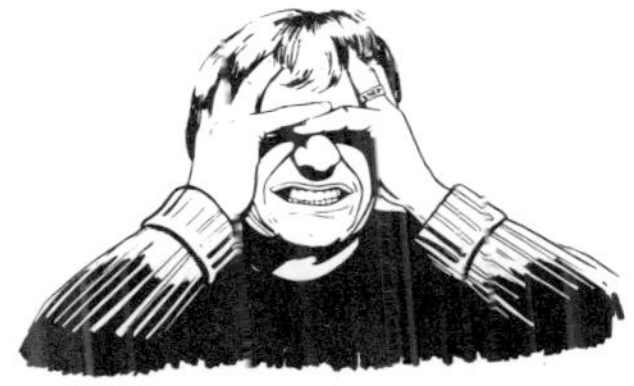

| Dehydration | Large fluid load |
|---|---|
| 1. High | Low |
| 2. Osmoreceptors | Osmoreceptors |
| 3. Stimulated | Suppressed |
| 4. Increased | Decreased |
| 5. Large | Small |
| 6. Small | Large |
| 7. High | Low |

## Frame 19

There are also some other factors that can affect ADH secretion.

Stresses such as anxiety, severe pain, and emotional disturbances can override osmotic stimuli and cause secretion of ADH and retention of water.

Some beta-adrenergic stimulators such as isoproterenol HCl (Isuprel) increase ADH release. Opiates and barbiturates can have the same effect.

Jane Wilson is in ICU following an auto accident. She has a number of broken bones, severe lacerations, and bruises, and is being evaluated for internal injuries. The other victims of the crash did not survive. She is receiving 3,000 ml/day of balanced IV solution but her urinary output is 600 ml of concentrated urine. Her eyelids look puffy. Assuming that her renal function is normal, why might she be retaining fluid?

Anxiety, severe pain, grief, and opiate drugs may be increasing ADH secretion and water conservation.

# Frame 20

Summary:

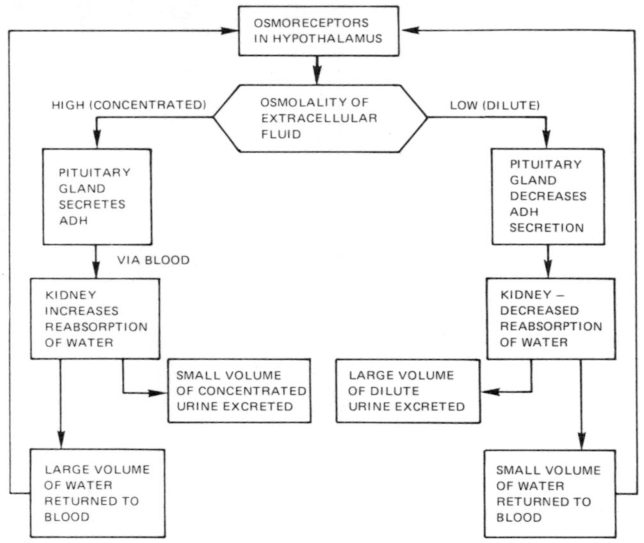

# PART IV IMPAIRMENT OF CONCENTRATION AND DILUTION MECHANISMS

## Frame 21

The urinary volume can vary from as little as 400 ml/day to as much as 3 liters/day, depending on the person's state of hydration.

With maximum ADH stimulation, the normal kidneys can concentrate the urine to 1,200 mOsm/kg.

With maximum ADH suppression, the urine can be diluted to 50 mOsm/kg.

True or False:

1. ______ Changes in a patient's extracellular sodium concentration would affect renal excretion of water.
2. ______ ADH causes the kidneys to excrete more water.
3. ______ A urine osmolality of 50 mOsm means that 50 osmotically active particles are dissolved in a unit volume of urine.
4. ______ Normal urine osmolality is a fixed value.
5. ______ Urine volume varies according to age, time of day, and diet.

1. True
2. False
3. True
4. False
5. True

## Frame 22

In renal disease the kidney's ability to reabsorb water and excrete concentrated urine is often impaired. Here are some reasons for lack of concentrating ability, which occurs in various renal diseases:

Decreased ability to reabsorb water and sodium in the proximal tubule

Impaired tubular ability to remove chloride and sodium in the Loop of Henle (Refer to Panel 1.) If less electrolyte is present in the interstitial space of the nephron, there is less osmotic pull on water in the distal tubule.

Loss of tubular sensitivity to ADH

Structural damage to cells that renders them incapable of reabsorbing water

1. The outcome of each of these factors would be (high/low) volume of urine output.
2. The (proximal/distal) tubule reabsorbs two thirds of the water in the filtrate?
3. If the tubules were not sensitive to ADH, a large volume of water would be (saved/excreted).
4. If a patient has defective concentration ability, (dehydration/water intoxication) would be expected.

Answers:

1. high
2. proximal
3. excreted
4. dehydration (The patient would lose a large volume of water.)

The patient with a concentrating defect may have azotemia, even though his urine volume is large. The urine osmolality is low with relatively few particles of nitrogenous waste excreted.

## Frame 23

In advanced chronic renal disease, the kidney may also lose the ability to dilute the urine and thereby excrete excess water. The precise mechanisms are not clearly understood but may involve

Increased ADH secretion due to low blood volume, low cardiac output, stress or narcotic drugs

Very reduced glomerular filtration rate with little water available for excretion

Inability of the tubule cells to reabsorb sodium and thus generate electrolyte-free water.

1. If a patient's kidneys were not able to dilute the urine, his intake of fluids would need to be (decreased/increased).
2. Defects in the ability to dilute the urine would lead to (dehydration/edema).

Answers:

1. decreased
2. edema

## Frame 24

The amount of water excreted by the kidney tubules can be increased by the action of diuretics. The thiazides, furosemide (Lasix) and ethacrynic acid (Edecrin) all inhibit the reabsorption of sodium and water in the tubules. As you noted while studying Panel 1, less sodium in the nephron's interstitial space results in less osmotic pull to reabsorb water from the distal tubule. Less sodium in the extracellular fluid will also reduce the amount of extra fluid held in that compartment.

1. Diuretics can be administered to renal patients to increase the (concentrating/diluting) capacity of the nephron.
2. After the administration of a potent diuretic like furosemide, the urine osmolality would be (increased/decreased).

1. diluting
2. decreased

## Frame 25

Which of these problems is reflected by each sign or symptom?

a. Loss of ability to concentrate urine
b. Loss of ability to dilute urine

1. ______ Nocturia (voiding during the night)
2. ______ No change in urine volume to match increases in intake
3. ______ Edema
4. ______ Urine output significantly greater than fluid intake

1. a (Normally the kidney concentrates urine at night.)
2. b (Increased intake should cause increased output.)
3. b (Excess fluid isn't being excreted in dilute urine.)
4. a (Fluid intake and output is usually in balance.)

## Frame 26

Here are some more terms and their definition:

*Anuria* refers to the inability of the kidney to produce urine, with a daily urine output of 0–100 ml. This results in no excretion of waste products of metabolism, extra electrolytes, or excess water.

*Oliguria* is the production of less than 400 ml urine per day.

*Polyuria* is the excretion of abnormally large amounts of urine which are usually dilute.

True or false:

1. ______ If a patient is anuric, the serum will contain a higher than normal amount of metabolic waste.

   1. True

2. ______ Polyuria is not harmful because waste products are excreted.

   2. False (Lots of water is lost, but waste products may be retained in renal failure.)

3. ______ A patient excreting 300 ml urine per day has oliguria.

   3. True

## Frame 27

Summary:

Depending on the state of hydration

1. Urine volume can vary from 400 ml to 3 liters/day.
2. Urine osmolality can vary from 1,200 to 50 mOsm/kg.

In renal disease the kidney's ability to concentrate urine can be impaired, causing polyuria, nocturia, dehydration, and urine osmolality fixed within 50 mOsm of plasma osmolality.

In advanced renal disease the ability to dilute urine may also be impaired, causing fixed urine volume and osmolality regardless of increased intake, edema, and fluid overload.

# CHAPTER 8
# ASSESSMENT: BODY FLUID BALANCE

This chapter reviews the clinical tests that assess kidney regulation of body fluids and physical signs of body water shifts.

After completing this chapter you will be able to

1. Given urine osmolality values, label them concentrated or dilute, and compare urine with serum osmolality
2. Differentiate between specific gravity and osmolality of urine in relation to what is measured, range, accuracy, and changes in renal failure
3. Correlate fluid balance with rapid changes in weight and urinary output data
4. Choose signs and symptoms indicating water loss or retention.

### Chapter outline

- Laboratory tests
    - Serum osmolality
    - Urine osmolality
    - Specific gravity of urine
- Physical signs
    - Weight
    - Intake and output
    - Dehydration
    - Fluid overload

# PART I
# LABORATORY TESTS

In Chapter 7 you saw that osmolality of interstitial fluid and serum are in equilibrium. Changes in serum osmolality affect osmotic pressure and fluid movement between fluid compartments. Remember, also, that the osmolality of extracellular fluid activates secretion of ADH. This hormone helps regulate the amount of water excreted by the kidney.

## Frame 1

*Serum* osmolality is kept quite constant at 290 ± 5 milliosmols per kilogram (mOsm/kg), however, the range of serum osmolality is

| Dilute | Normal | Concentrated |
|---|---|---|
| 260 | 290 ± 5 | 320 |

*Urine* osmolality is measured as dilute or concentrated in comparison to the serum osmolality levels:

| Dilute | Normal | Concentrated |
|---|---|---|
| 50 | 290 ± 5 | 1,200 |

Use this information to compare urine and serum osmolality.

1. The dilute urine has (more/less) particles than serum of normal osmolality.
2. The concentrated urine has (more/less) particles than serum of normal osmolality.

1. less
2. more

## Frame 2

In the following situations identify the urine osmolality as concentrated or dilute:

1. Don has been working for 7 hours in the hayfields on a hot day. He has not had access to much drinking water. His urine osmolality would perhaps be 320 mOsm/kg.
2. Saturday night Don relaxed at the local pub. He managed to put away two six-packs of beer. Now his urine osmolality would be about 120 mOsm/kg.

1. Concentrated
2. Dilute

3. At a picnic supper on Sunday, Don ate many salty foods including chips, dill pickles, and hot dogs with catsup and mustard. His urine osmolality now would be about 750 mOsm/kg.

3. Concentrated

In chapter 7 you also learned about the role of ADH in response to extracellular osmolality.

Review this response.

**Frame 3**

1. If the serum osmolality is 320 mOsm/kg, more water needs to be (excreted/saved).
2. This would (stimulate/inhibit) the secretion of ADH.
3. The urine excreted would have a (high/low) osmolality.

1. saved
2. stimulate
3. high

**Frame 4**

1. If the serum osmolality is 270 mOsm/kg, more water needs to be (excreted/saved).
2. This (inhibits/stimulates) the secretion of ADH.
3. The urine excreted would have a (high/low) osmolality.

1. excreted
2. inhibits
3. low

**Frame 5**

Decide what happened to the serum osmolality and ADH secretion in each situation:

| | *Serum osmolality* | *ADH secretion* |
|---|---|---|
| Situation 1: Dehydration | Increased/ Decreased | Stimulated/ Inhibited |
| Situation 2: High fluid intake | Increased/ Decreased | Stimulated/ Inhibited |
| Situation 3: High sodium intake | Increased/ Decreased | Stimulated/ Inhibited |

| *Serum osmolality* | *ADH secretion* |
|---|---|
| 1. Increased | Stimulated |
| 2. Decreased | Inhibited |
| 3. Increased | Stimulated |

*Panel 1*

***In renal failure the kidney loses its diluting and concentrating ability. The urine osmolality and specific gravity are two methods of assessing urine concentration.***

| *Specific Gravity of Urine* | *Osmolality of Urine* |
|---|---|
| *1. Depends on number, size and weight of dissolved particles* | *1. Depends on total number of dissolved particles regardless of size or weight* |
| *2. Range 1.001–1.025 g/ml compared to distilled water, which has a specific gravity of 1 g/ml* | *2. Wider range of normal, 50–290–1,200 mOsm/kg, because it is compared to serum osmolality* |
| *3. False high readings if high molecular weight particles are present: glucose, protein, mannitol, x-ray dyes* | *3. More accurate information, not affected by size and weight of particles* |
| *4. In renal failure the specific gravity reflects the tubules' inability to dilute or concentrate. In some situations the value stays at 1.010 regardless of fluid regulation needs.* | *4. As the kidney loses diluting and concentrating ability, the urine osmolality will stay within 50 mOsm of the serum osmolality.* |

## Frame 6

Mr. Johnson is admitted to ICU for observation after an anaphylactic reaction to IVP dye.

His urine output is being monitored every 2 hours. The specific gravity is also checked. Over the past 12 hours the specific gravity has been rising (1.019 to 1.032) although urine output has remained steady at an average of 40 ml/hour.

Refer to Panel 1 when answering these questions:

1. Does x-ray dye have a high or low molecular weight?
2. What has this done to the specific gravity of Mr. Johnson's urine?
3. Is specific gravity a good way to assess Mr. Johnson's renal function?

1. High
2. False high reading
3. No

## Frame 7

Glucose, protein, and mannitol are also particles of high molecular weight.

1. Would their presence in urine increase or decrease its specific gravity? This would be considered a false reading.
2. How does the molecular weight of glucose affect the specific gravity of a diabetic who has glucosuria?
3. If the patient has no glycosuria or proteinuria, would the specific gravity be roughly equivalent to the osmolality?

1. Increase
2. The specific gravity would be high.
3. Yes (The normal particles in urine: urea, Na, Cl, and K, are of low molecular weight.)

## Frame 8

1. Is the most accurate method of assessing the concentrating and diluting capacity of the kidney by determining osmolality or specific gravity?
2. Why?

1. Osmolality (If you answered specific gravity, review Frames 6 and 7.)
2. The size and weight of particles influence specific gravity. Large molecules such as glucose and protein give false high readings.

## Frame 9

Tests of the kidney's concentrating ability are altered when the patient is taking diuretics.

1. A diuretic medication (increases/decreases) water output.
2. The patient's urine should be (concentrated/dilute).
3. Urine osmolality (will/will not) demonstrate kidney response to a diuretic drug.

1. increases
2. dilute
3. will

## Frame 10

Urine osmolality is considered dilute or concentrated in comparison with serum osmolality. Remember, the glomerular filtrate is about the same osmolality as plasma, and most of the water is normally reabsorbed by the tubules. As the kidney loses its concentrating ability in renal failure, much of the water is left in the filtrate and the urine osmolality becomes fixed within 50 mOsm of serum:

| *Serum* | *Filtrate* | *Urine* |
|---|---|---|
| 290 mOsm | 290 mOsm | 300 mOsm |

Mark these statements true or false:

1. ______ When concentrating ability is lost, the serum, filtrate, and urine have about the same amount of dissolved particles per unit volume.
2. ______ Normally, much water would be reabsorbed from the filtrate by the tubules, making urine osmolality higher than serum osmolality.
3. ______ If urine osmolality becomes fixed near the serum osmolality, the kidney tubules are not efficient in changing the composition of the filtrate to meet the body's needs.

1. True
2. True
3. True

## Frame 11

Mrs. Harris is 60 years old. She's dehydrated due to vomiting and diarrhea. Her specific gravity on the routine admission urinalysis is 1.007.

1. This specific gravity is (dilute/concentrated).
2. In a dehydrated person, serum osmolality would (increase/decrease).
3. This should stimulate the kidney to (save/excrete) fluid.
4. With normal kidney function, the urine should become (concentrated/dilute).
5. Mrs. Harris (should/should not) be evaluated for renal failure.

If she does have renal failure, her dehydration would be corrected more slowly to avoid complications such as pulmonary edema.

1. dilute
2. increase
3. save
4. concentrated
5. should

## Frame 12

Mrs. Bonn is 47 years old. She has had recurring pylonephritis over the past 10 years. The specific gravity of her urine on a morning specimen is 1.023.

1. Is this a normal specific gravity?

2. Basing your decision on this fact alone, does she have renal damage due to the recurring pyelonephritis?

1. Yes (The kidney will concentrate the urine during sleep.)

2. No

## Frame 13

Summary:

Normal serum osmolality is 290 ± 5 mOsm/kg.

Chief osmotically active particles are sodium, glucose, and urea.

Changes in serum osmolality cause ADH levels to increase or decrease.

Normal urine osmolality (mOsm/kg) range is

| Dilute | Normal | Concentrated |
|---|---|---|
| 50 | 290 ± 5 | 1,200 |

Urine specific gravity range is 1.001–1.025 g/ml.

Specific gravity measures the number, size, and weight of dissolved particles, while osmolality measures number only. Specific gravity gives false high readings if high molecular weight particles are present in urine, for example, glucose, protein, mannitol, x-ray dyes.

In renal failure

Urine osmolality is fixed within 50 mOsm of serum level.

Urine specific gravity reflects the kidney's inability to respond to changes in fluid needs of the body.

# PART II PHYSICAL SIGNS

## Frame 14

You've completed the discussion of lab tests that should be assessed in following the kidney's control of fluid balance. Now look at the physical findings.

The two most important measures are the patient's daily weight, and fluid intake and output balance.

A patient who gains more than 1 lb per day is thought to be retaining fluid. One pound is equivalent to about 500–600 ml of fluid. (A liter of fluid will be reflected by a gain of about 1 kg.)

1. A patient who gains 4 lb in 1 day would have retained about how much fluid?
2. One kilogram is equivalent to how many liters of fluid?
3. One pound is equivalent to how many ml of fluid?

Answers:

1. 2,000 ml, or 2 liters
2. 1 liter
3. 500–600 ml

## Frame 15

To control excess retention of fluid, a patient in renal failure is limited to 500 ml intake plus the amount of output from the previous day. The 500 ml replaces the insensible losses of fluid (respiratory, skin, GI).

1. If Mrs. Jones' output yesterday was 600 ml, how much intake can she have today?
2. Mr. Olson is anuric. What should his daily intake total?

Answers:

1. 1,100 ml
2. 500 ml/day

Fluid intake for the critically ill patient may be based on hourly urine output and be replaced ml for ml.

*Panel 2*
*Physical Signs of Fluid Loss and Gain*

*Fluid Loss*

*Early signs*
*Weight loss of ½ lb a day, weakness, dizziness, exhaustion, irritability, thirst*

*Signs of severe loss*
*Dry mucous membranes, poor skin turgor, fever, cool extremities, postural hypotension, increased pulse*

*Fluid Retention*

*Early signs*
*Weight gain; edema of fingers, ankles, and around eyes; increased blood pressure*

*Signs of rapid fluid gain*
*Disorientation, weakness, twitching, nausea, vomiting, headache, blurred vision, muscle cramps, shortness of breath, increased respiration, moist rales, chest pain, increased CVP, neck vein distention*

**Frame 16**

This is Mrs. Jones' 4th day in acute renal failure which resulted from hemorrhagic shock after a bowel resection. Her weight has increased from 148 to 150 lb since yesterday. Her past 24-hour urinary output was 400 ml, and intake was 1,500 ml.

1. Is Mrs. Jones losing or retaining water?
2. Which of these signs and symptoms could you expect today?
   a. Sacral edema
   b. Dyspnea
   c. Pinched skin stands in dry peaks
   d. Rales
   e. A fixed urine osmolality

1. Retaining
2. a, b, d, e

## Frame 17

Mrs. Harris, who has renal failure complicated by diarrhea, is dehydrated. Choose the symptoms she might have:

a. Thirst
b. Weakness
c. Tachycardia
d. Edema
e. Postural hypotension (orthostatic)

a, b, c, e

## Frame 18

Mr. Benson is on chronic hemodialysis. His weekly urine output is less than 100 ml but dialysis will remove the excess fluid. He is to limit his fluid intake to 500 ml per day.

This past weekend Mr. Benson went to a family gathering and had gained 6 lb by the time of his next dialysis. Which of these signs and symptoms might you expect him to have?

a. Orthostatic hypotension
b. Hypertension
c. Dyspnea
d. Chest pain

b, c, d

## Frame 19

Mrs. Rice is also on chronic hemodialysis. Toward the end of today's dialysis, she became hypovolemic because too much fluid was removed.

What signs or symptoms would she exhibit?

a. Orthostatic hypotension
b. Tachycardia
c. Weakness
d. Hypertension

a, b, c

## Frame 20

List the data the nurse needs to assess a patient's fluid balance:

| Lab Data | Physical Observations |
|---|---|
| ______________ | ______________ |
| ______________ | ______________ |
| | ______________ |
| | ______________ |

| Lab Data | Physical Observations |
|---|---|
| Serum osmolality<br>Urine osmolality or specific gravity | Weight<br>Fluid intake and output<br>Vital signs<br>Signs of dehydration or overload |

## Frame 21

Summary:

One pound of body weight is equivalent to about 400–600 ml fluid.

One kilogram of body weight is equivalent to about 1 liter fluid. Insensible losses of fluid are about 500 ml/day.

In renal failure fluid may be restricted to 500 ml/day; or in a critically ill patient it may be replaced according to hourly output.

Signs of fluid overload are weight gain, decreased urine volume, edema, dyspnea, rales.

Signs of dehydration are weight loss, hypotension, tachycardia, weakness, poor skin turgor, thirst, fever.

# CHAPTER 9

## BODY BUFFERING MECHANISMS

The metabolic processes of the body generally produce excess acid. The lungs and kidneys are involved in regulating the amount of acid and base in body fluids within a narrow range. The role of the kidney in this process is the subject of this chapter. When you are finished with this chapter you will be able to

1. Explain the importance of maintaining acid-base balance
2. Recognize a buffering system in the body
3. Recognize two chief mechanisms of hydrogen ion excretion by the kidney
4. List the two main functions of the kidney in maintaining acid-base balance
5. Explain the role of the lungs in maintaining acid-base balance
6. Contrast the kidney's buffering system in acidosis and alkalosis
7. Given kidney impairments in buffering ability, predict the systemic outcome.

### Chapter outline

Review of Fundamental Concepts
- Acid
- Base
- pH

Buffers
- Definition
- Action of buffers in the body

Renal response to acidemia
- Elimination of excess hydrogen ion
- Restoration of bicarbonate
- Effects of inadequate response

Renal response to alkalemia
- Excretion of hydrogen ion
- Excretion of bicarbonate
- Factors hindering this response

# PART I REVIEW

The material in this chapter deals with the acid and alkaline compounds in the body. Briefly review some chemistry.

## Frame 1

An acid is a compound that releases a hydrogen ion when in a solution with water.

Hydrochloric acid (HCl) is a compound found in the body. If added to water, this is what it does:

$$HCl \longrightarrow H^{+} + Cl^{-}$$

The $H^{+}$ is a hydrogen ion.

True or false:

1. _____ If a large amount of acid is added to water, a small number of hydrogen ions will be released.
2. _____ To find out if a solution is acidic, you could measure the concentration of hydrogen ions.
3. _____ Acids are hydrogen ion donors in solution.

Answers:

1. False
2. True
3. True

## Frame 2

A base is a compound that accepts a hydrogen ion into its molecular structure when in a solution with water.

Bicarbonate ($HCO_3^-$) is an important compound in the body. When in a solution with water, this is what it does:

$$HCO_3^- + H^{+} \longrightarrow H_2CO_3$$

1. A base is a proton (donor/acceptor) in solution.
2. In an alkaline (basic) solution, the concentration of free hydrogen ions is (high/low).

Answers:

1. acceptor
2. low (The base combines with the available hydrogen ions.)

## Frame 3

The following phrases describe the properties of acids and bases. Write "acid" or "base" in front of each, depending on which term the phrase describes.

1. ______ Hydrogen ion acceptor — 1. Base
2. ______ Releases hydrogen ions in an aqueous solution — 2. Acid
3. ______ Incorporates hydrogen ions into its molecular structure by removing them from solution — 3. Base

## Frame 4

One way to measure acidity and alkalinity—or hydrogen ion concentration of solutions—is with pH.

Because of the mathematical calculations involved, pH is inversely related to hydrogen ion concentration.

If the hydrogen ion concentration is *high,* pH is *low* and the solution is *acid.*

If the hydrogen ion concentration is *low,* pH is *high* and the solution is *alkaline.*

Blood pH is precisely regulated between 7.35 and 7.45.

Complete these statements about blood pH:

1. A blood pH of 7.30 indicates excess (acid/base). — 1. acid
2. A high blood pH means that there are (more/fewer) hydrogen ions, and that the blood is (acid/alkaline). — 2. fewer alkaline

Excess acid in the blood is called *acidemia,* while excess base is called *alkalemia.* In each example of pH, indicate whether the blood is

a. Acidemic
b. Alkalemic
c. Normal

1. ______ 7.40 — 1. c
2. ______ 7.47 — 2. b
3. ______ 7.23 — 3. a
4. ______ 7.30 — 4. a

## Frame 5

Mark these statements true or false:

1. ______ The pH is a measurement of hydrogen ion concentration in a solution.
2. ______ An acid solution has a high pH value.
3. ______ If a patient's blood pH is 7.5, he or she is alkalemic.

1. True
2. False
3. True

## Frame 6

The most important acid in the body is carbonic acid ($H_2CO_3$), and the most important base is bicarbonate ($HCO_3^-$).

The metabolic processes of the body produce an excess of acid. Therefore, large amounts of base are needed to balance the solution. This figure shows the relationship of amounts of acid and base and pH.

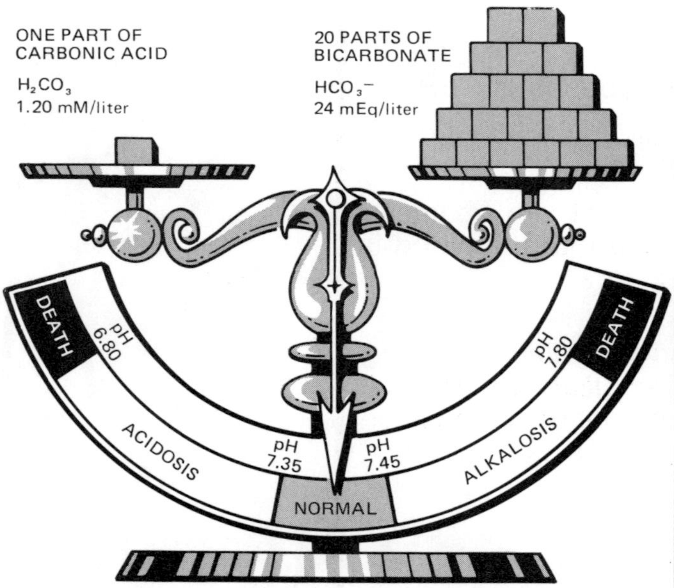


Figure 43

If the proportion of carbonic acid and bicarbonate change, the pH changes. For example, if 10 parts of bicarbonate are removed, the pointer would swing toward 7.10 on the acidosis side.

1. If the amount of bicarbonate increases, pH moves toward (acidosis/alkalosis).

   1. alkalosis

2. If the pH were 7.0, the acid content would probably be (higher/lower) than the normal proportion.

   2. higher

3. If a patient had only 10 parts of bicarbonate available, the pH would indicate (acidosis/alkalosis).

   3. acidosis

4. pH is (directly/inversely) related to hydrogen ion concentration.

   4. inversely

5. The metabolic processes predispose the body toward (acidosis/alkalosis).

   5. acidosis (Metabolism of protein results in a large load of acid by-products.)

# PART II BUFFERS

## Frame 7

The chemical environment of the cell is crucial for maintaining normal function. One of the most important factors is the amount of acid in the cell and tissue fluids. There is a very narrow range within which cell enzymes can function to carry on life processes.

If less than 1/40,000 of the daily acid by-products were to remain free in the blood, death would rapidly occur. However, a highly efficient system is used to trap the hydrogen ions immediately as they enter the extracellular fluid, and to remove them from the body.

A buffer is a chemical compound that acts like a chemical sponge. It can "soak up" extra hydrogen ions or release them to prevent fluctuations in the pH. The buffer system is the first line of defense until the lungs and kidneys can excrete excess acid or base.

1. If a large amount of acid is present in the blood, what will the buffer system do regarding hydrogen ions?

   1. Take up hydrogen ions

2. A patient has a significant excess of base in his blood. What will the buffers do?

   2. Release hydrogen ions

3. Define buffer in your own words.

   3. Did you include these ideas? Compound that can take up excess hydrogen ions in an acid solution or release hydrogen ions if base is predominant, in order to maintain the correct acid-base ratio

4. What organs assist the buffers in regulating acid-base balance?

   4. Lungs, kidneys

## Frame 8

Now look at how specific buffers in the body prevent or minimize a drastic change in pH when strong acids are added to the blood.

An example of a buffer pair is carbonic acid ($H_2CO_3$) and sodium bicarbonate ($NaHCO_3$). As you can see in the figure, hydrogen ions from protein metabolism combine with the bicarbonate ion ($HCO_3^-$) to form carbonic acid ($H_2CO_3$). This dissociates into water and carbon dioxide.

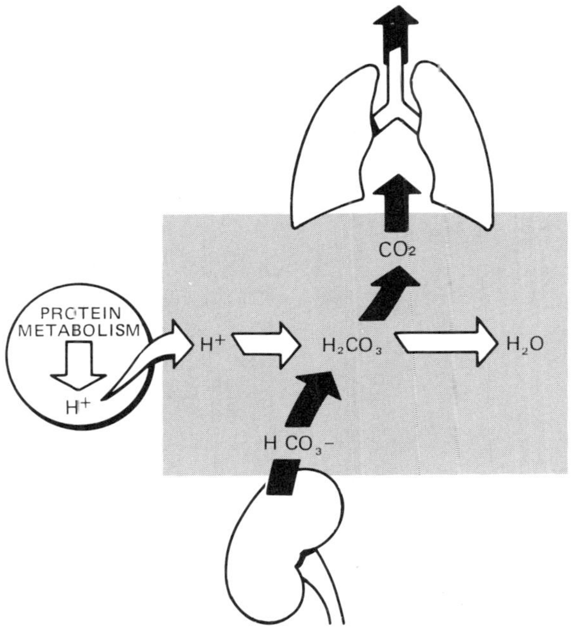


Figure 44

Neal S. Bricker, ed., *The Sea Within Us.* N.Y.; Science and Medicine Publ. Co., Inc. 1975, p. 38.

1. What organ of the body eliminates most of the $CO_2$?
2. What organ supplies the bicarbonate?
3. Would the reserve supply of bicarbonate available to buffer excess acid be increased or decreased by this reaction?

1. Lung
2. Kidney
3. Decreased, as the available bicarbonate combines with hydrogen ions (The kidneys continually reabsorb bicarbonate to replenish the supply.)

## Frame 9

You have already seen that cell metabolism results in acid by-products, which must be neutralized and excreted.

The body cells themselves have a buffering effect—red blood cells and even bone cells are buffers. Alone, this would not be enough to buffer metabolic acids.

So the plasma buffers, primarily carbonic acid and bicarbonate, are crucial in maintaining the narrow range of blood pH in the face of the acid load from metabolism of foods.

1. Are waste products from the metabolism of foods acid or alkaline?
2. If the plasma had no buffers, what would happen to the blood pH value?
3. Why must the pH range in the blood be so carefully maintained?

1. Acid
2. It would go down.
3. Cell enzymes are not able to function well out of the range. Cell death can result.

## Frame 10

Summary:

The physiologic processes of the body usually produce an excess of acid.

The body must rid itself of excess acid to maintain pH in the normal range: 7.35–7.45 which is crucial to cellular processes.

The first line of defense against imbalance is circulating buffer compounds. Buffers are compounds that can absorb excess hydrogen ions or release them to maintain the pH of a solution.

The most important buffer pair is carbonic acid and sodium bicarbonate. Bicarbonate combines with hydrogen ions produced by metabolism, forming carbonic acid, which dissociates into carbon dioxide and water. Carbon dioxide is then excreted by the lungs.

# PART III RENAL RESPONSE TO ACIDEMIA

## Frame 11

An ordinary diet results in an acid excess of about 50 mEq of hydrogen ion ($H^+$) daily. When this is added to the blood, the plasma buffer reaction takes place.

Choose the correct words in parentheses, indicating what happens when the buffer reaction occurs.

1. There is (increased/decreased) production of carbon dioxide gas.
2. There is (raising/lowering) of the bicarbonate level.

1. increased
2. lowering

Despite the lungs' excretion of carbon dioxide, there are still excess hydrogen ions in the blood. The role of the *kidney,* then is to

Eliminate the excess hydrogen ion

Replenish the bicarbonate level in the blood.

Are plasma buffers able to combine with all of the acid produced during metabolism?

No

## Frame 12

*Elimination of excess hydrogen ions*

In the distal tubule hydrogen ions combine with a phosphate buffer in the filtrate ($HPO_4^=$) to form phosphoric acid ($H_2PO_4$) for excretion.

| Capillary | Tubule cells | Filtrate in tubule lumen |
|---|---|---|
| | $H^+$ ⟶ | $HPO_4^=$ ↓ $H_2PO_4$ (Excreted) |

The tubule cells can make ammonia from amino acids in response to low blood pH. The ammonia ($NH_3$) combines with hydrogen ions to become the ammonium ion ($NH_4^+$). It is secreted in combination with chloride as a neutral salt.

| Capillary | Tubule cells | Filtrate in tubule lumen |
|---|---|---|
| Glutamine | $NH_3$ + $H^+$ → | $NH_4^+ + Cl^-$ (Excreted) |

These two buffer systems allow for elimination of hydrogen ions without making the urine so acid that it would damage the tissues.

1. Do phosphate and ammonia release or combine with hydrogen ions?
2. Hydrogen ion is excreted in combination with what two compounds?
3. Why is it important that the hydrogen ions be buffered before being excreted in the urine?

1. Combine with
2. Phosphate, ammonia
3. A highly acid urine could damage cells.

## Frame 13

*Restoration of bicarbonate*

The second function of the kidney is to replenish the bicarbonate level. This is a continuous operation in the nephron.

- • The proximal tubule cells reabsorb almost all of the bicarbonate filtered by the glomerulus.
- •• The tubule excretes hydrogen ($H^+$) in exchange for sodium ($Na^+$). This reabsorbed sodium then combines with the reabsorbed bicarbonate to form the sodium bicarbonate buffer.

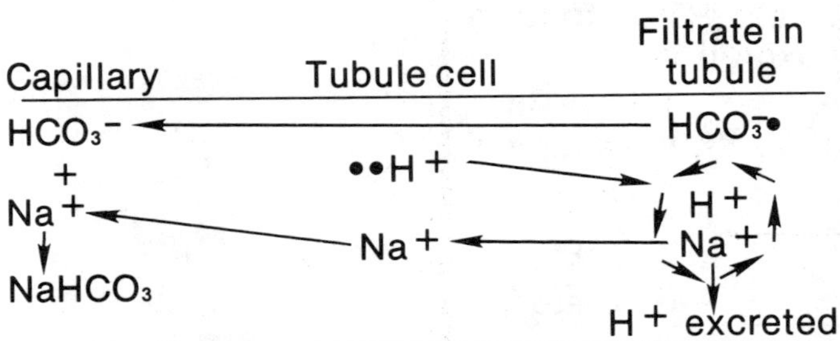


1. The kidney ____________ filtered bicarbonate.
2. The kidney also reabsorbs ____________ to combine with bicarbonate to form the buffer.

1. reabsorbs
2. sodium

3. The two functions of the kidney in regulating acid-base balance are __________ and __________.

3. excrete excess hydrogen ions
   replenish bicarbonate level

## Frame 14

*Effects of inadequate response*

Sometimes the normal body defenses against acidosis can be overwhelmed. Mr. Harris has severe acidosis due to acute renal disease. Because of an infectious renal disease, the glomerular membranes of 90% of his nephrons are fibrotic and unable to function in filtration. Since the filtration surface is so drastically reduced, metabolic waste products such as uric acid, urea, and creatinine build up in the blood.

1. True or False:
   a. ______ Given enough time, Mr. Harris' plasma buffers will combine with the excess hydrogen ions and bring the pH back to normal.
   b. ______ The kidney tubules will act to compensate by excreting more hydrogen ions with ammonia and phosphates.
   c. ______ The lungs will not be of any aid in getting rid of excess acid.

1.
   a. False (Plasma bicarbonates have probably been depleted, since the patient is in acidosis.)
   b. True, if the tubules are unaffected by disease
   c. False (The lungs will blow off extra $CO_2$ with fast and deep respiration.)

2. You would expect (high/low) blood pH, (high/low) level of bicarbonates in the blood, and (high/low) BUN.

2. low
   low
   high

## Frame 15

Summary:

The kidney tubules excrete excess hydrogen ions in exchange for sodium.

The hydrogen ion is excreted in combination with phosphate and ammonia buffers.

The sodium is reabsorbed to replenish the sodium bicarbonate buffer compound.

The kidneys restore the bicarbonate level in the blood by reabsorbing bicarbonate and sodium.

# PART IV RENAL RESPONSE TO ALKALEMIA

## Frame 16

So far, you have learned about how the kidneys protect the body against excess acidity. Next, look at what happens when body fluids become too alkaline.

Mr. Davidson had severe and prolonged nausea and vomiting, and lost much hydrochloric acid in the emesis.

Choose the correct words in parentheses, indicating effects of the significant loss of body acid:

1. Mr. Davidson's blood pH would be (lower/ higher) than normal.
2. The normal ratio of acid to base would be changed with (more base present/more acid present).

1. higher

2. more base present

## Frame 17

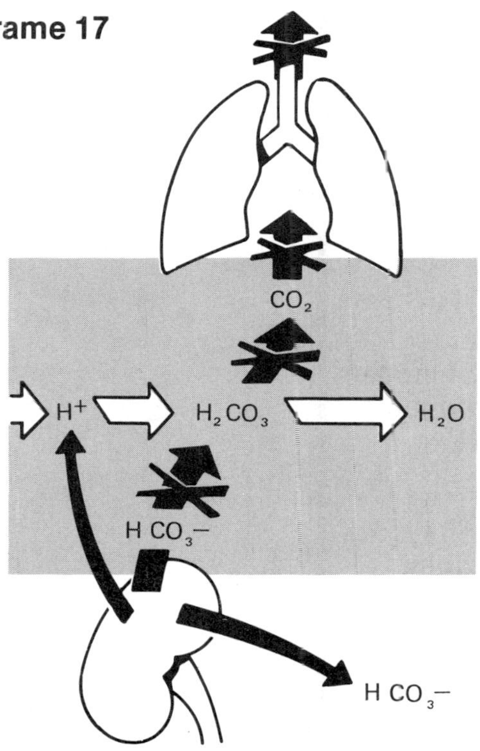


Figure 45

To make up for Mr. Davidson's loss of acid

The lungs decrease the rate and depth of respirations, thereby blowing off less $CO_2$. This slows the dissociation of carbonic acid into $CO_2$ and water, thereby, increasing the acid content of the blood.

The kidneys return more hydrogen ions to the blood rather than excreting them in the urine, and bicarbonate is excreted rather than reabsorbed.

Refer to the figure when selecting the correct words.

1. The purpose of the compensation mechanisms is to (increase/decrease) the amount of carbonic acid in the blood.
2. Carbonic acid (is/is not) part of a buffer compound.
3. The combined effect of lungs and kidneys in this situation would be to (raise/lower) blood pH.

1. increase
2. is
3. lower

## Frame 18

This system of compensation for excess alkalinity can also be hindered.

Potassium deficiency within the cells (caused by loss of potassium in emesis and no oral intake of the ion) can influence the kidney to save bicarbonate instead of excreting it.

Dehydration (from emesis and lack of intake) can stimulate sodium—and bicarbonate—reabsorption.

True or false:

1.______ Cellular potassium deficiency can influence renal compensation of alkalosis.

2.______ Fluid balance is unrelated to renal buffering mechanisms.

1. True
2. False

## Frame 19

> Summary:
>
> In alkalosis, the kidney increases the carbonic acid content of the blood by
>
> 1. Reabsorbing hydrogen ions
> 2. Excreting bicarbonate
>
> The lungs increase carbonic acid levels by decreasing the rate and depth of respirations, thus reducing the excretion of carbon dioxide.

## Frame 20

In both acidosis and alkalosis the respiratory system is the first to compensate. If the change in carbon dioxide removal is not adequate after several hours, the kidneys will begin to compensate also.

Fill in the blanks, describing what happens when the blood becomes acidotic or alkalotic:

1. If the blood is becoming acidotic, first the lungs will __________________, then the kidneys will save__________________ and excrete ______________.

1. blow off more $CO_2$ by increasing rate and depth of respiration, bicarbonate, hydrogen ions

2. If the blood is becoming alkalotic, first the lungs will __________________, then the kidneys will save__________________ and excrete ______________.

2. retain $CO_2$ by hypoventilation, hydrogen ions, bicarbonate

## Frame 21

1. If the kidney tubules' ability to regulate acid-base balance were impaired by disease, which of the following would you expect?

1. a, b, d
(c is done by the lungs.)

a. Decreased formation of ammonia in the tubules
b. Change in ability to excrete and save hydrogen ions
c. Reduced excretion of carbon dioxide gas
d. Inability to reabsorb bicarbonate

2. If the kidney tubules were unable to form ammonia, excrete hydrogen ions, and reabsorb bicarbonate, what would happen to the blood pH?

2. pH would decrease resulting in acidosis.

# CHAPTER 10

# ASSESSMENT: BODY BUFFERING MECHANISMS

A number of parameters are valuable in assessing the kidney's role in acid-base balance. At the conclusion of this chapter you will be able to

1. Evaluate pH values
2. Differentiate between $CO_2$ content, $P_{CO_2}$, and base excess measurements
3. Identify the cause for variation in urine pH
4. Recognize the clinical picture of acidosis.

## Chapter outline

Serum pH

Measures of alkaline reserve
  $CO_2$ content
  Base excess

Urine pH

Clinical picture of acidosis

# PART I
# SERUM pH

## Frame 1

There are several lab tests that help with assessing the body's state of acid-base balance in patients with renal disease. They are the pH, $HCO_3$, and base excess of arterial blood gases; venous $CO_2$ content; and urinary pH.

Normals

| | | |
|---|---|---|
| Arterial pH | = | 7.35-7.45 |
| $HCO_3$ | = | 21-29 mEq/liter |
| Base excess | = | 0 ± 2 U |
| $CO_2$ content | = | 22-30 mEq/liter |
| Urinary pH | = | average 6.0 (4.6-8.0 depending on diet) |

Ms. Larson has normal renal function. What is the kidney's function in relationship to hydrogen ions and bicarbonate:

1. Hydrogen ions are (reabsorbed/excreted).
2. Bicarbonate is (reabsorbed/excreted).

1. excreted
2. Reabsorbed

## Frame 2

In renal failure the kidney loses its ability to regulate acid-base balance.

Choose the conditions under which metabolic acidosis can occur:

a. Decreased ability of the tubule to excrete $H^+$ ions
b. Decreased formation of ammonia in the tubule
c. Decreased ability of the tubule to reabsorb bicarbonate
d. Decreased serum pH due to dietary restriction of protein

a, b, c (Dietary restriction of protein would not contribute to metabolic acidosis.)

(If you need review, see Chapter 9, Frames 11-13 and 21.)

## Frame 3

Mr. Brown has renal failure secondary to chronic glomerulonephritis. On admission his arterial pH was 7.30.

1. The serum pH level becomes (higher/lower) with acidosis due to renal failure.
2. This change in serum pH would indicate (an increased/a decreased) serum bicarbonate level and (more/less) hydrogen ions in the blood.
3. Why does the body maintain a critical blood pH range?

(For review, see Chapter 9, Frame 7.)

1. lower
2. decreased
   more
3. Cell enzymes are not able to function out of the range.

# PART II MEASURES OF ALKALINE RESERVE

## Frame 4

*Venous* $CO_2$ content should not be confused with the $P_{CO_2}$ of *arterial* blood gases.

$CO_2$ content measures the alkali reserve of the body which is primarily bicarbonate. (normal = 22–30 mEq/liter)

$P_{CO_2}$ is the pressure (tension) of dissolved $CO_2$ gas in the blood—influenced only by the lungs.

Mrs. Rice, who has chronic glomerulonephritis, is acidotic with a serum pH of 7.32. In a first attempt to correct the acidosis, her respiratory rate will increase to eliminate more $CO_2$ gas. Then available bicarbonate in the blood will be used to buffer the excess acid. But, her kidneys are not normally efficient in restoring bicarbonate to the blood and excreting excess acid.

1. If $CO_2$ content reflects the amount of bicarbonate available to buffer acids, would Mrs. Rice's $CO_2$ content be high or low?

1. Low (The bicarbonates are being used up and are not being replenished.)

2. Which of these values would be closest to her $CO_2$ content: 18.0 mEq/liter or 34.0 mEq/liter?

2. 18.0 mEq/liter

3. What is $CO_2$ content?

3. It is the measurement of the alkali reserve of the body, which is primarily bicarbonate.

## Frame 5

Base excess (BE) is another method of assessing the severity of acid-base imbalances. A normal base excess is 0 ± 2 U. For example, + 7 means there is an excess of alkali (base), while -9 would mean an excess of acid. The number is calculated considering all alkali reserves including serum proteins, such as hemoglobin, which also act as buffers.

1. Mrs. Rice's BE is −3. This means she has (excess/normal/no excess) base.
2. Mr. Brown's BE is +6. He has (excess/normal/no excess) base.
3. Ms. Larson's BE is +1. She has (excess/normal/no excess) base.

1. no excess
2. excess
3. normal

# PART III
# URINE pH

## Frame 6

Urine pH is normally acid, about 6.0. Normal kidneys can respond to dietary changes and acid-base imbalances by producing urine with pH ranging from 4.5 to 8.0.

1. Choose the correct words in parentheses to complete these statements relating to respiratory acidosis:
   a. If a patient is retaining $CO_2$ because of poor lung function, he can become acidotic. If the kidneys are normal, they will (increase/decrease) hydrogen ion excretion.
   b. More hydrogen ions in the urine would (raise/lower) urinary pH.

2. Now complete these statements relating to metabolic acidosis due to renal failure:
   a. If a patient's kidney tubules are unable to function normally, (more/less) hydrogen ion can be secreted in the urine, and less bicarbonate is reabsorbed.
   b. In this case, the urinary pH would be (more alkaline/more acid).

Some organisms causing urinary tract infections will alter the pH of urine. Certain medications can also have this effect.

1.
   a. increase
   b. lower (More acidic)

2.
   a. less
   b. more alkaline

# PART IV CLINICAL PICTURE OF ACIDOSIS

## Frame 7

Metabolic acidosis can be recognized by physical symptoms as well as by laboratory evidence of depleted bicarbonate reserve and an acidic pH. Respiratory compensation, central nervous system depression, and weakness may be apparent.

Choose the signs and symptoms of metabolic acidosis:

a. Serum pH = 7.42
b. $CO_2$ content = 18 mEq/liter
c. Lethargic
d. Increased rate and depth of respirations
e. Base excess of −4 U

b, c, d, e

## Frame 8

Mrs. Rice, the patient with chronic glomerulonephritis, has a respiratory rate of 30 deep breaths per minute (Kussmaul's respiration). She is restless but difficult to wake.

Choose the lab data you would expect with this situation:

a. pH = 7.28
b. $HCO_3$ = 24 mEq/liter
c. $CO_2$ content = 12 mEq/liter
d. $HCO_3$ = 14 mEq/liter
e. Base excess = +7 U

a, c, d

## Frame 9

Summary:

To evaluate the acid-base balance in patients with kidney disease, consider the following factors:

Serum pH is usually acidic due to retention of acid metabolic wastes, and inability to excrete $H^+$ and to reabsorb bicarbonate.

These parameters are usually low due to failure to reabsorb bicarbonate:

$HCO_3$

$CO_2$ content

Base excess

Urinary pH is usually alkalotic due to excretion of bicarbonate and lack of hydrogen ion excretion.

Normal values for these tests are

Serum pH = 7.35–7.45
$HCO_3$ = 21–29 mEq/liter
Base excess = 0 ± 2 U
$CO_2$ content = 22–30 mEq/liter
Urinary pH = 6

Physical signs of acidosis include the following: Kussmaul's respiration as the lungs compensate for acidosis by blowing off more $CO_2$; central nervous system depression with confusion, lethargy or coma.

# Section 3

# Case Studies: Acute Renal Problems

# INTRODUCTION TO SECTION 3

*This section of the book is organized around case studies of three patients with renal disease. This will give you an opportunity to apply to patient care situations what you learned in Sections 1 and 2.*

*In order to simulate the clinical situation more closely, we will use another method of programming in this section. It will allow you to confront a large amount of information and select the appropriate factors, to explore the relationships between the factors, and to use your creativity and decision-making ability. This method is called "structural communication," and here is a brief example.*

It is the year 1992. You are working in a computerized critical care unit. You have continuous access to a large amount of information about each of your patients. The response indicator below lists some of the available information. Use it to construct solutions to the following problems.

*Problem 1*

What information would you request to monitor the patient's fluid balance? Squares numbered: ____________

*Problem 2*

If your patient was retaining fluid, which of these values would progressively increase? Squares numbered: ____________

| Response Indicator | | | |
|---|---|---|---|
| CVP 1 | Arterial $O_2$ 2 | ECG pattern 3 | Hourly urine output 4 |
| Arterial blood pressure 5 | Blood pH 6 | Hourly IV infusion volume 7 | $CO_2$ content 8 |
| Serum creatinine 9 | Urine osmolality 10 | Body weight 11 | Pulse rate 12 |

*Next you will compare your answers with the suggested responses. Explanations are then given about the most important factors which must be included and those which are clearly wrong. This is the system for alerting you to these key factors:*

| Response Indicator | | | |
|---|---|---|---|
| CVP 1 | Arterial $O_2$ 2 | ECG pattern 3 | Hourly urine output 4 |
| Arterial blood pressure 5 | Blood pH 6 | Hourly IV infusion volume 7 | $CO_2$ content 8 |
| Serum creatinine 9 | Urine osmolality 10 | Body weight 11 | Pulse rate 12 |

*Problem 1* — Fluid Balance

Suggested Responses: 4, 7, 10, 11

O [4, 7, 10, 11> *(Means: If you OMITTED 4, 7, 10 or 11, read this comment, to see why these factors are essential)*

Hourly urine output compared with the hourly intake (via IV infusion) gives an estimate of fluid balance. Urine osmolality would show whether the kidneys are saving or excreting water, and body weight changes will reflect fluid losses and gains.

I [1, 3, 5, 12> *(Means: If you INCLUDED 1, 2, 4, or 12 read this comment)*

If you included these because fluid imbalances often affect cardiovascular function, you were correct. However these parameters are not direct measurements of fluid balance as are the suggested responses.

I [6, 8>

These values measure acid-base balance rather than fluid balance.

I [9>

Measures clearance of metabolic waste rather than fluid balance.

*Problem 2* — Fluid Retention

Suggested Responses: 1, 5, 11, 12

O [1, 5, 12>

Increased blood volume increases the pressure in the arteries (the arterial blood pressure) as well as the venous system (central venous pressure). The pulse rate will also rise as the heart increases its rate to pump the higher volume of blood.

O [11>

Remember that retention of 500-600ml of water will be reflected by a gain of about one pound of body weight.

I [4, 7, 10>

If the patient is retaining fluid his urinary output could be lower than normal, or it could be rising progressively but not keeping pace with the need to excrete water. The osmolality may decrease as more water is excreted, or it may be higher than normal if the kidneys are not able to dilute the urine effectively. The fluid overload may be caused by an increased IV infusion volume. But it may be due to cardiovascular or electrolyte problems with no change in intake.

*In the comment section the most troublesome wrong answers will be discussed, as well as the most important correct answers. You may come up with some combinations that did not occur to us, or that show a broad understanding of the relationships between factors. This also reflects the reality of clinical practice: there are many ways to identify relevant information and to solve problems.*

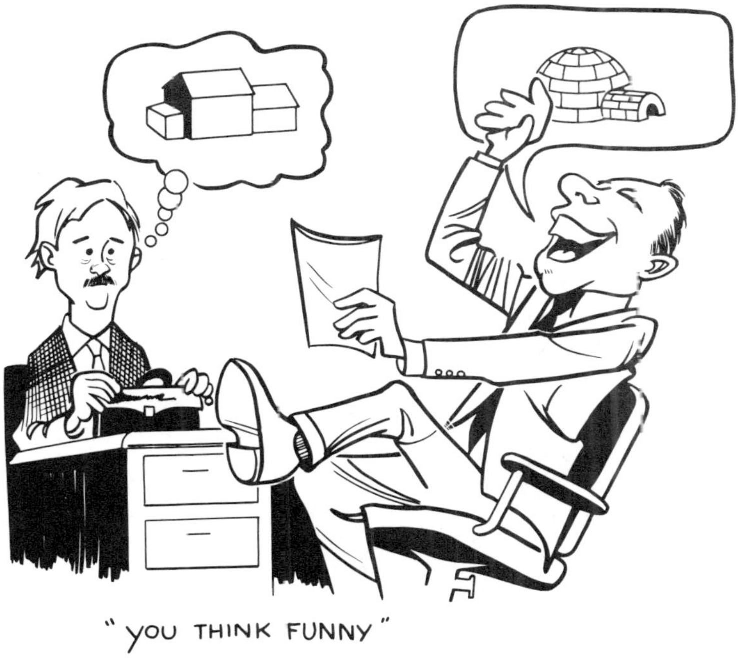

# CHAPTER 11

# END-STAGE RENAL DISEASE

## INTRODUCTION

Chronic renal failure usually involves a gradual loss of functioning nephrons. At the beginning of this process, the body compensates for the loss of nephrons; and the patient has few, if any, symptoms. As the disease progresses and destroys more nephrons, the patient experiences more and more systemic symptoms. When most of the nephrons are damaged and the glomerular filtration rate drops below 10 ml/min, the patient is considered to have end-stage renal disease.

This chapter illustrates the progressive nature of renal failure with the case of Suzanne Rice. Upon completion of the chapter you will be able to

1. Describe the typical clinical picture of chronic progressive renal disease
2. Review the medical management of chronic renal disease
3. Identify factors important in making a nursing assessment
4. Develop a nursing care plan for a patient in end-stage renal failure.

## CASE PRESENTATION

### Beginning of the Disease Process

Suzanne Rice grew up on a farm and attended a small town school. At age 10 she developed a sore throat during an epidemic of strep throat in her school. Six days after the sore throat began, Suzanne's eyes and ankles were puffy and her urine was a reddish brown. Her parents brought her to their doctor who noted, "entire body is edematous, hematuria present." She was hospitalized immediately. Urine output was about 400 ml/day. Urinalysis showed gross hematuria and 4+ proteinuria. Her hemoglobin (Hgb.) was 10 g. Her blood pressure was 150/104.

The doctor's diagnosis was acute poststreptococcal glomerulonephritis. Suzanne was put on bed rest and a low-salt diet. She received magnesium sulfate to prevent seizures from the elevated blood pressure.

Within 7 days, Suzanne's output was greater than 1,500 ml/day. She had lost 7 kg (15 lb) of weight. Urinalysis showed microscopic hematuria and 1+ to 2+ albuminuria. Her blood pressure was 120/90. She was sent home on restricted activity and kept out of school for the remainder of the winter.

Following this episode, Suzanne did not require any medical care, as she was in good health.

### Diminished Renal Reserve

At age 21 Suzanne was married, and a year later she became pregnant. Prenatal exams showed that she had trace to 1+ proteinuria, and her blood pressure began to rise. Her blood pressure was controlled with dietary salt and water restriction. She delivered a normal healthy child without further problems.

Normal kidneys have more than enough reserve capacity to handle the additional demands caused by pregnancy. In Mrs. Rice's case, it can be seen that there were not quite enough functioning nephrons to handle increased needs.

### Renal Insufficiency

Over the next 3 years Mrs. Rice began to notice that she tired very easily and was extremely fatigued at the end of the day. She had swollen ankles by evening, and noticed that her wedding ring was uncomfortably tight. During a routine visit to her gynecologist the doctor noted 2+ albuminuria and a blood pressure of 154/96. After reviewing her history he decided to refer Suzanne to the nearby renal clinic for a thorough evaluation of her renal status. Many diagnostic tests were performed, including a kidney biopsy.

This showed a specimen with seven glomeruli. Each had evidence of sclerosing and hyalinizing. (Hyalin is a substance found in degenerated cells.) There was narrowing of the arterioles. An immune process was suggested by the deposit of immune complexes along the endothelial side of the basement membrane.

Recall that antibodies formed against streptococci can become "confused" and attack normal membranes in the kidney, damaging the cells. The biopsy results suggest that this autoimmune response was the cause of Mrs. Rice's progressive loss of nephrons.

## DISCUSSION

In the first part of the book, you learned about the effects of renal disease on major kidney function, and you reviewed methods of measuring renal function. Now you will use structural communication to describe the typical clinical picture of chronic progressive renal disease.

*Problem 1*

The symptoms and diagnostic data found during Mrs. Rice's evaluation are presented on the Response Indicator. Find the data that you think reflect problems with body protein homeostasis.
Squares numbered: ____________

*Problem 2*

Now choose the data showing problems with solute reabsorption and excretion. Squares numbered: ____________

*Problem 3*

What data reflect the renal tubule's declining ability to regulate body fluid balance? Squares numbered: ____________

Now check your answers under Comments, which follows the Response Indicator.

| Response Indicator | | | |
|---|---|---|---|
| Blood urea nitrogen (BUN): 45 mg/100 ml (n = 8–20) 1 | Serum creatinine (Scr): 2 mg/100 ml (n = 0–1.0) 2 | Creatinine clearance (Ccr): 13.5 ml/min average to 15% (n = 85–125) 3 | Serum phosphorus ($PO_4$): 5.8 mg/100 ml (n = 2.45–4.5) 4 |
| Serum calcium (Ca): 8.2 mg/100 ml (n = 8.5–10) 5 | Hemoglobin: 9.8 g (n = 12–16) Hematocrit: 32/100 ml (n = 38–54) 6 | Serum sodium (Na): 143 mEq/L (n = 135–145) 7 | Serum potassium (K): 4 mEq/L (n = 3.6–5.5) 8 |
| Serum albumin: 2.5 g/100 ml (n = 3.2–5.6) 9 | Urine specific gravity: 1.009 (morning specimen) (n = 1.001–1.025) 10 | Nocturia: 1 or 2 times/night 11 | Urine pH: 6 (n = 4.8–8.5) 12 |
| Urine volume: 1,500 ml/24 hr (average) (n = 600–2500) 13 | Blood pressure: 150/90 (average) 14 | Weight gain: 12 lb (5.4 kg) in 2 months 15 | Fluid intake: 1,900 ml/24 hr (average) 16 |
| Proteinuria: 2+ 17 | | | |

| Response Indicator | | | |
|---|---|---|---|
| Blood urea nitrogen (BUN): 45 mg/100 ml (n = 8–20) 1 | Serum creatinine (Scr): 2 mg/100 ml (n = 0–1.0) 2 | Creatinine clearance (Ccr): 13.5 ml/min average to 15% (n = 85–125) 3 | Serum phosphorus ($PO_4$): 5.8 mg/100 ml (n = 2.45–4.5) 4 |
| Serum calcium (Ca): 8.2 mg/100 ml (n = 8.5–10) 5 | Hemoglobin: 9.8 g (n = 12–16) Hematocrit: 32/100 ml (n = 38–54) 6 | Serum sodium (Na): 143 mEq/L (n = 135–145) 7 | Serum potassium (K): 4 mEq/L (n = 3.6–5.5) 8 |
| Serum albumin: 2.5 g/100 ml (n = 3.2–5.6) 9 | Urine specific gravity: 1.009 (morning specimen) (n = 1.001–1.025) 10 | Nocturia: 1 or 2 times/night 11 | Urine pH: 6 (n = 4.8–8.5) 12 |
| Urine volume: 1,500 ml/24 hr (average) (n = 600–2500) 13 | Blood pressure: 150/90 (average) 14 | Weight gain: 12 lb (5.4 kg) in 2 months 15 | Fluid intake: 1,900 ml/24 hr (average) 16 |
| Proteinuria: 2 + 17 | | | |

## Comments

Remember:

| | | | |
|---|---|---|---|
| I | 4 or 6 | MEANS: | If you included in your response 4 or 6, read this comment. |
| O | 5 | MEANS: | If you omitted 5 in your response, read this comment. |

*Problem 1* — Protein Homeostasis

Suggested responses: 6, 9, 15 and 17.

O 6

Hemoglobin is made from protein. When the pool of body protein is low, less hemoglobin is formed, as in Suzanne's case.

The kidney also produces erythropoietin, a hormone that stimulates red blood cell production. Kidney disease interferes with production of this hormone, and anemia is the result. The life span of the red blood cell is also shortened in uremia, so as the disease progresses one would expect even more severe anemia.

O 9, 15, 17

Protein is leaking out of the plasma through the damaged glomerular membrane and into the urine. So there is low serum albumin and proteinuria. Less protein in the plasma results in decreased osmotic pull in the vascular space. This causes fluid to move into the interstitial space, causing edema. This fluid shift is reflected in the weight gain. If you are still unclear about this, you may wish to review Chapter 3, Frames 16–22.

I 4, 5, 7, 8

These values show the kidney's ability to reabsorb electrolytes from the filtrate, which are needed to maintain normal blood levels, and to excrete excess electrolytes. There is probably no relationship to protein homeostasis.

I 10

If you were thinking about how the presence of protein in the urine can affect specific gravity, you might have included this one. Actually, proteinuria causes a false high specific gravity reading, so Suzanne's urine osmolality would be a more accurate measurement. Neither of these is helpful in assessing protein homeostasis, however.

I 1, 2, 3

The retention of the nitrogenous wastes from protein metabolism could also be considered a problem of protein homeostasis.

| Response Indicator | | | |
|---|---|---|---|
| Blood urea nitrogen (BUN): 45 mg/100 ml (n = 8-20) 1 | Serum creatinine (Scr): 2 mg/100 ml (n = 0-1.0) 2 | Creatinine clearance (Ccr): 13.5 ml/min average to 15% (n = 85-125) 3 | Serum phosphorus ($PO_4$): 5.8 mg/100 ml (n = 2.5-4.5) 4 |
| Serum calcium (Ca): 8.2 mg/100 ml (n = 8.5-10) 5 | Hemoglobin: 9.8 g (n = 12-16) Hematocrit: 32/100 ml (n = 38-54) 6 | Serum sodium (Na): 143 mEq/L (n = 135-145) 7 | Serum potassium (K): 4 mEq/L (n = 3.6-5.5) 8 |
| Serum albumin: 2.5 g/100 ml (n = 3.2-5.6) 9 | Urine specific gravity: 1.009 (morning specimen) (n = 1.001-1.025) 10 | Nocturia: 1 or 2 times/night 11 | Urine pH: 6 (n = 4.8-8.5) 12 |
| Urine volume: 1,500 ml/24 hr (average) (n = 600-2500) 13 | Blood pressure: 150/90 (average) 14 | Weight gain: 12 lb (5.4 kg) in 2 months 15 | Fluid intake: 1,900 ml/24 hr (average) 16 |
| Proteinuria: 2+ 17 | | | |

*Problem 2* — Solute Reabsorption and Excretion

Suggested responses: 1, 2, 3, 4, 5

O 2 or 3

Creatinine is a waste product of metabolism which is normally almost completely cleared from the blood by the kidneys. Therefore it is a very accurate measure of the kidney's ability to excrete wastes. It can be seen that creatinine is building up in Suzanne's blood as the rate of clearance drops to 15% of normal.

O 1

BUN tends to rise if the kidney is not efficient in clearing urea from the blood. But, if you omitted this because a high dietary intake of protein may also cause increased BUN, you were on the right track. Urea is a much less accurate measure of clearance. However, in view of the creatinine clearance and other data, you could assume that Suzanne's elevated BUN is due to renal problems.

O 4 or 5

Notice that the serum $PO_4$ is elevated as the nephrons lose their capacity to excrete excess phosphorus. The calcium is low due to decreased dietary intake and tubular inability to absorb enough calcium to keep blood levels normal. Because of this disturbance in the ratio of calcium and phosphorus, Suzanne could have problems with bone demineralization. If you need to review kidney function in balancing these electrolytes, refer to Chapter 5, Frames 15–22.

I 7 or 8

Serum sodium and potassium are within the range of normal, so wouldn't be considered a problem at this point. The sodium level is at the high end of the range. Some patients with renal disease have hypernatremia because excess water in the extracellular fluid triggers the release of aldosterone and reabsorption of more sodium. Some renal patients have hyponatremia because their kidneys are unable to reabsorb enough sodium.

| Response Indicator | | | |
|---|---|---|---|
| Blood urea nitrogen (BUN): 45 mg/100 ml (n = 8-20) 1 | Serum creatinine (Scr): 2 mg/100 ml (n = 0-1.0) 2 | Creatinine clearance (Ccr): 13.5 ml/min average to 15% (n = 85-125) 3 | Serum phosphorus ($PO_4$): 5.8 mg/100 ml (n = 2.45-4.5) 4 |
| Serum calcium (Ca): 8.2 mg/100 ml (n = 8.5-10) 5 | Hemoglobin: 9.8 g (n = 12-16) Hematocrit: 32/100 ml (n = 38-54) 6 | Serum sodium (Na): 143 mEq/L (n = 135-145) 7 | Serum potassium (K): 4 mEq/L (n = 3.6-5.5) 8 |
| Serum albumin: 2.5 g/100 ml (n = 3.2-5.6) 9 | Urine specific gravity: 1.009 (morning specimen) (n = 1.001-1.025) 10 | Nocturia: 1 or 2 times/night 11 | Urine pH: 6 (n = 4.8-8.5) 12 |
| Urine volume: 1,500 ml/24 hr (average) (n = 600-2500) 13 | Blood pressure: 150/90 (average) 14 | Weight gain: 12 lb (5.4 kg) in 2 months 15 | Fluid intake: 1,900 ml/24 hr (average) 16 |
| Proteinuria: 2+ 17 | | | |

*Problem 3* — Fluid Balance

Suggested responses: 10, 11, 13, 14, 15, 16

O 13, 14, 15, 16

When you look at the relationship between intake, output and weight gain, you see that Suzanne is retaining excess fluid in the interstitial compartment. This shows the kidney's inability to precisely regulate fluid balance. The blood pressure may also rise as water is retained in the vascular compartment.

O 10 or 11

Normal kidneys produce a small amount of concentrated urine at night. Suzanne's morning specimen is dilute, and she needs to void during the night. This shows that her kidneys are beginning to lose their ability to concentrate urine.

I 6, 9, 17

The loss of protein indicated by the values does contribute to shifts of water between fluid compartments. However, the heavy loss of protein occurs in the glomerulus. This problem focused on the *tubular* functions such as concentration and dilution of urine.

# CASE PRESENTATION

## Medical Management

Mrs. Rice was discharged from the renal clinic on this medical regimen:

*Diet*

40 g of high biologic value protein (essential amino acids) and 4–6 g sodium.

Metabolism of a restricted protein diet should result in less urea, and the sodium restriction could decrease the amount of sodium and water retained by the kidney.

The 40 g of essential protein allowed in the diet will help maintain the serum albumin and hemoglobin level. However, Suzanne will need to eat foods totaling about 2,500 calories each day to prevent the burning of body protein for energy.

*Diuretic*

Furosemide (Lasix) 60 mg/day. This drug increases renal excretion of water by inhibiting sodium reabsorption by the tubules. Due to increased water excretion, the plasma and interstitial fluid volume would be decreased. This drug may cause depletion of potassium, so Suzanne should be watched for hypokalemia.

*Phosphorus binder*

Aluminum hydroxide (i.e. Amphojel) taken with each meal to bind phosphorus in the GI tract, thus lowering the serum phosphorus. The excess phosphorus is eliminated in the feces. Dioctyl sodium sulfosuccinate (Colace) is used to counteract the constipating effect of aluminum hydroxide by its stool-softening action.

## Renal Failure

Mrs. Rice continued on this program of medical management for the next 2½ years. Although the doctors warned her that the kidney damage might progress, Suzanne hoped that the signs and symptoms were only temporary and that the medical plan would restore her health. But as time went on, she began to have frequent headaches, nausea, and vomiting. At night she was bothered by muscle cramps, aches, and twitching, and by a frequent need to void. She was losing weight and her blood pressure was rising steadily. The furosemide dosage was increased and a hypotensive agent, methyldopa (Aldomet) (250 mg t.i.d.), was begun. A solution of sodium citrate and citric acid was prescribed to correct metabolic acidosis. This weak acid solution is converted to bicarbonate by the liver.

Mrs. Rice continued to manage her household, even though she felt ill due to all the symptoms mentioned. In addition, her kidneys were no longer producing enough erythropoietin—a hormone that stimulates development of red blood cells. This caused anemia. Suzanne also found that she felt drowsy, apathetic, and unable to concentrate for long periods.

These symptoms were depressing and discouraging. Mrs. Rice felt that she was a failure as a wife and mother, she became irritable and impatient, and she found it difficult to maintain her family relationships.

Mrs. Rice acknowledged the fact that she needed dialysis when she could not walk up the stairs because of weakness in her legs, and when she hired household help. The smallest task would leave her physically and mentally exhausted. Five years after kidney problems had first been diagnosed, Mrs. Rice was admitted to the hospital in end-stage renal failure.

About two weeks prior to the admission a simple arteriovenous fistula was surgically created during an outpatient visit to provide access to circulation for hemodialysis treatments.

Suzanne's first hospital day was taken up with diagnostic tests. This chart shows that her renal function had deteriorated significantly:

| | Blood test | Previous | Present | Normal | |
|---|---|---|---|---|---|
| Clearance of wastes | BUN | 45 | 112 | 8–20 | mg/100 ml |
| | Creatinine | 2 | 9.8 | 0–1 | mg/100 ml |
| | Creatinine clearance | 13.5 | 5.7 | 85–125 | ml/min |
| Electrolytes | Potassium | 4 | 5 | 3.6–5.5 | mEq/liter |
| | Phosphorus | 5.8 | 7 | 2.45–4.5 | mg/100 ml |
| Acid-base balance | pH | — | 7.33 | 7.35–7.45 | |
| | $CO_2$ content | — | 17.5 | 24–30 | mEq/liter |

*Urinalysis*

| | |
|---|---|
| Specific gravity | 1.010 |
| Proteinuria | 3+ |
| RBCs | 40–50 |

In addition an intravenous pyelogram showed that both kidneys were small, with severely decreased function. The renogram showed extremely slow flow, excretion, and clearance of radioactive material from both kidneys. Nerve conduction studies revealed a mild slowing of motor conduction in the right and left peroneal nerves. This was consistent with the degree of neuropathy.

To determine the medical plan of care, the physicians considered the elevated serum levels of nitrogen wastes in spite of a controlled diet, the nausea and vomiting, the uncontrolled hypertension, the diminished nerve conduction velocities, and the minimal renal blood flow. These factors indicated that Mrs. Rice should begin dialysis without delay. Plans were begun for peritoneal dialysis as her simple fistula was still underdeveloped.

Ellen Fredericks was asked to be Mrs. Rice's primary nurse. The assessment she made soon after Suzanne's admission follows.

## Admission Assessment Form — Chronic Renal Failure

Name *Suzanne Rice*

Admission Date *2/27*

Age *27* Sex *F*

Religion *Protestant*

Marital Status *Married*

Children (ages) *5 (daughter)*

Height *5′6″*

Weight: Present *116*

Usual *122*

T *98°* P *72* R *16*

BP: Supine *164/112* AP: Supine *72*

Standing *120/90* Standing *78*

---

1. Renal—Urinary Output
   - a. Color *dark yellow*
   - b. Amount *a pint a day*
   - c. X Nocturia ___Burning X Frequency ___Distention ___Urgency ___Retention ___Pain X Foamy

2. Cardiac
   - a. See BPs above
   - b. Irregular pulse *no*
   - c. Pericardial friction rub *no*
   - d. Other abnormal heart sounds ___
   - e. Chest pain *no*
   - f. Pulsus paradoxus ___
   - g. Other: *dizzy when she stands up rapidly*

3. Body Fluids
   - a. See weights above
   - b. Edema:

     ___Slight X Feet X Sacrum
     X Moderate X Ankles ___Abdomen
     ___Pitting ___Legs ___Periorbital

4. Respiratory
   - a. Rate *16* b. Depth ___
   - c. Odor ___
   - d. Breathing difficulties

     Dyspnea: ___Bedrest X Walking—*2 blks.* ___Sitting X Stairs
     ___Cheyne Stokes ___Kussmaul
     ___Other: ___
   - e. Cough: ___Moist ___Hacking ___Productive
   - f. Lung sounds: X Clear ___Rales ___Moist ___Wheezes

5. Neural
   - a. Mental status: ___Alert ___Confused X Drowsy ___Comatose ___Inattentive X Forgetful

     ___Other: *unable to concentrate on what's said—fell asleep*
   - b. Orientation to time, place, person *ok*

5. Continued
   - c. Sensory disturbances: ___Visual ___Olfactory ___Auditory ___Tactile
   - d. Motor disturbances:

     Gait (difficulty walking) ___
     Tingling ___
   - e. Other *headaches, esp. a.m.*

6. Gastrointestinal
   - a. Mouth X Dry ___Ulcers
   - b. Appetite: *"poor"*

     X Anorexia X Nausea X Vomiting
     Best meal *lunch*
   - c. X Indigestion ___Diarrhea ___Pain X Constipation X Hiccups ___Blood in stool ___Coffee-ground emesis

7. Skin
   - a. Color *dark tan*

     ___Pallor ? Jaundice
     ___Cyanotic ___Gray brown
     X Pruritus X Bruises
     ___Lesions ___Crystals
     X Dryness
   - b. Perspiration:

     Increased___ Normal___ Decreased___

8. Musculoskeletal
   - a. Muscles: X Good tone ___Flaccid

     ___Atrophy *thin* ___"Renal flap"
     X Cramps *at night, along with aches and twitching*
     Other: *legs so weak I can't climb stairs*
   - b. Skeletal: ___Pain ___Fractures

9. Endocrine

   ___Delayed puberty ___Decreased potency
   X Decreased libido
   ___Amenorrhea

10. Behavior on admission

    ___Apprehensive/anxious X Discouraged
    ___Restless/agitated X Withdrawn
    ___Irritable X Depressed
    ___Demanding ___Calm
    ___Other: ___

## DISCUSSION

When Mrs. Rice is treated with dialysis, some of her problems will be significantly improved. Dialysis will remove excess water and edema will subside. This will also cause improvement in her blood pressure. Waste products of metabolism and other toxins will be removed. This will bring her electrolyte balance into normal range and also improve the alterations in sensory, perceptual, and cognitive functioning. Acidosis will also be corrected. (In following chapters, you will study dialysis and the nursing care required.)

Mrs. Rice will continue to have a number of other problems that require nursing intervention. You know quite a bit about Suzanne Rice, now. Considering her diagnostic data, admission assessment, and other information, use the Response Indicator to identify nursing problems which are important in planning her current care.

*Problem 1*

Choose the factors that contribute to Mrs. Rice's nutritional problem. Squares numbered: ____________

*Problem 2*

Choose the factors contributing to Mrs. Rice's problem with maintaining a healthy balance between activity and rest. Squares numbered: ____________

*Problem 3*

Choose the factors that Mrs. Rice needs to understand in order to manage her self-care requirements in the future. Squares numbered: ____________

*Problem 4*

Which factors contribute to Mrs. Rice's need for assistance in coping psychologically with her situation? Squares numbered: ____________

| Response Indicator | | | |
|---|---|---|---|
| Impairment of urinary elimination and alteration of patterns 1 | Alteration of bowel elimination 2 | Prevention of respiratory and cardiovascular complications 3 | Protein deficiency 4 |
| Denial of illness 5 | Impairment of skin integrity 6 | Low level of energy and strength 7 | Fear of hospitalization and treatment procedures 8 |
| Alterations in body image 9 | Altered sexual functioning 10 | Depression 11 | Nausea, anorexia 12 |
| Impairment of family and other social relationships 13 | Pain or discomfort 14 | Less mobility (due to bone demineralization and neuropathy) 15 | Anemia 16 |

| Response Indicator | | | |
|---|---|---|---|
| Impairment of urinary elimination and alteration of patterns 1 | Alteration of bowel elimination 2 | Prevention of respiratory and cardiovascular complications 3 | Protein deficiency 4 |
| Denial of illness 5 | Impairment of skin integrity 6 | Low level of energy and strength 7 | Fear of hospitalization and treatment procedures 8 |
| Alterations in body image 9 | Altered sexual functioning 10 | Depression 11 | Nausea, anorexia 12 |
| Impairment of family and other social relationships 13 | Pain or discomfort 14 | Less mobility (due to bone demineralization and neuropathy) 15 | Anemia 16 |

## Comments

*Problem 1* — Nutrition

Suggested responses: 1, 2, 4, 11, 12, 14 and 16

O 4, 16

The protein deficiency is at the basis of her nutritional problem. Lack of protein for cell repair and formation of enzymes hinders the metabolic work of cells. In anemic states less oxygen is delivered to the cells for metabolic activity. These factors cause all of the cells of the body to function at less than optimal levels.

O 1, 2

Because Suzanne's kidneys are unable to function adequately, her diet will need to be restricted so that fluid, electrolytes and metabolic wastes do not build up too rapidly between dialysis treatments.

Constipation is a problem that is also related to nutrition. Adequate bowel elimination must be established if any nutritional plan is to succeed.

O 11, 12, 14

Depression, nausea, and pain are all factors that would affect Suzanne's appetite and therefore her ability to cooperate with a nutritional plan.

I 7, 8, 9, 10, 13, 15

If you have included these because they may also affect appetite, you were correct.

I 3, 6

Complications such as respiratory infections and skin breakdown may occur more readily in a malnourished person. But because Suzanne does not have these problems now, they were not considered contributory to present nutritional problems.

*Problem 2* — Activity and Rest

Suggested responses: 1, 2, 4, 7, 11, 12, 14, 15, 16

O 1, 2, 4, 7, 12, 16

The problems of anemia and low energy levels are related to one another, as explained in Problem 1, and are a big part of this problem. The nutritional problems all relate to anemia and low energy and strength. Severe constipation can cause discomfort which deprives the patient of rest, and nocturia can interfere with sleep at night.

O 11, 14, 15

One of the characteristics of depression is a low activity level. Pain and discomfort would also limit Suzanne's activity as well as interrupt her rest. The decreased mobility is also contributory.

I 8, 9, 10, 13

If you included these factors because they would cause worry which would interfere with rest, you may be correct.

| Response Indicator | | | |
|---|---|---|---|
| Impairment of urinary elimination and alteration of patterns 1 | Alteration of bowel elimination 2 | Prevention of respiratory and cardiovascular complications 3 | Protein deficiency 4 |
| Denial of illness 5 | Impairment of skin integrity 6 | Low level of energy and strength 7 | Fear of hospitalization and treatment procedures 8 |
| Alterations in body image 9 | Altered sexual functioning 10 | Depression 11 | Nausea, anorexia 12 |
| Impairment of family and other social relationships 13 | Pain or discomfort 14 | Less mobility (due to bone demineralization and neuropathy) 15 | Anemia 16 |

*Problem 3* — Learning Needs for Self-Care

Suggested responses: 1, 2, 3, 4, 6, 7, 10, 13, 14, 15, 16

These are correct because Suzanne will need to understand the physical manifestations of her illness and ways to prevent and/or alleviate the symptoms. The psychological factors were not included here, as they are not considered learning needs for self-care. The psychological factors will, of course, affect Suzanne's readiness to learn and to manage her self-care.

*Problem 4* — Psychological Coping

Suggested responses: 7, 10, 11, and 13

O 7, 11

Suzanne's feelings of depression, as well as her low energy level, may hinder her ability to mobilize her personal resources to cope with illness.

O 10, 13

Prolonged illness tends to disrupt family relationships, social contacts, and recreational activities. This impairment of sexual and social relationships place an added stress on Suzanne. She may feel less able to rely on her husband, family, and friends for support.

I 5, 8, 9

Many patients with end-stage renal failure have these problems. Hospitalization and the extensive diagnostic testing can be frightening. Even more so is the complex dialysis procedure. Body image disturbances can arise from dependence on a machine for life, bodily changes due to uremia, and the appearance of the shunt. But, we did not find any evidence in the data presented that these were concerns for Suzanne. We think it is important to recognize that all patients don't have the same problems. It is good to keep these things in mind, however, since additional data may show that these are also problems for Suzanne.

# NURSING CARE PLAN: GOALS AND INTERVENTIONS

The next step is to identify goals and interventions that would be appropriate for Suzanne's problems.

## *Problem 1* — Nutrition

### Frame 1

Which of these goals (or outcomes) would you include on the care plan:

a. Normal serum protein
b. Normal hemoglobin
c. No complaints of nausea
d. No vomiting
e. Ability to eat most of food served
f. Regular bowel movements

c, d, e, f (If you included a and b, see Frame 2.)

### Frame 2

It is quite hard for the patient on a protein-restricted diet, who is nauseated, not hungry, and has other GI complaints, to attain a normal serum protein level. Anemia may continue because of the lack of erythropoietin and RBC destruction. This may be treated by giving anabolic steroids (such as testosterone) to build up red blood cell mass, by administering iron dextran (Imferon) and other medications to provide additional iron, and by dietary management. Sometimes blood transfusions are given for severe symptoms of anemia.

### Frame 3

Which of these approaches should be used to solve the nutritional problem?

a. Diet high in potassium and magnesium
b. Administration of antiemetic medications with individualized dosage pattern
c. Selective menu

b, c, d, e, f, h

d. Small, frequent meals
e. Pleasant surroundings and social interaction at mealtime
f. Oral hygiene before meals
g. Nothing by mouth until nausea subsides
h. Trial of laxatives and/or stool softeners to find the most effective kind and timing
i. Daily small nonirritating enemas

### *Problem 2* — Lack of Strength and Energy

### Frame 4

Choose the appropriate goal(s) for this problem at the predialysis stage of Suzanne's illness:

a. Ability to carry out self-care independently
b. Patient feels that her level of activity does not cause undue fatigue
c. Activity level increases each day

b

### Frame 5

Which of these interventions might help meet this goal?

a. Work out gradual activity plan with occupational therapy
b. Assist with personal hygiene
c. Encourage independence in self-care
d. Schedule frequent rest periods between procedures and activities
e. Eliminate annoyances such as noise and interruptions
f. Provide activities Suzanne was able to enjoy at home

b, d, e, f

Think for a moment about the nurse using *time* as an intervention modality. Timing is an important factor in the selection of nursing interventions. Remember that Suzanne is at the stage in her illness when the toxic effects of retained metabolites are causing severe physical and mental disabilities. Conservation of her energy is important now. After she goes on dialysis and begins to feel better, it will become important to encourage independence in self-care and to work out a graded activity plan. These interventions will later be crucial in Suzanne's rehabilitation.

## *Problem 3* — Learning Needs for Self-Care

### Frame 6

The effect of Suzanne's feelings on her readiness to learn has already been discussed. Consider also the effects of uremia on her alertness, ability to concentrate and to process information. Choose an appropriate goal related to her learning needs at this stage of her illness. b

a. Able to explain the most significant points about causes and effects of renal disease
b. Indicates satisfaction with answers to her questions and explanation of procedures
c. Demonstrates ability to perform simple self-care procedures
d. Expresses evidence of future planning regarding health care

### Frame 7

Since information giving to meet current needs seems most appropriate at this time, choose the best approaches Ellen can use to meet the goal: a, c, d

a. Willingness to repeat information as needed
b. Use anatomic models, charts, and patient education literature
c. Develop a trusting relationship with the patient by displaying competence, being available, and anticipating needs
d. Use brief, concrete, simple explanations so patient can give consent to procedures
e. Include Suzanne in group meetings for patient instruction and support

## *Problem 4* — Psychological Coping

### Frame 8

Feelings of depression are usually related to a significant loss. Suzanne has lost good health and all that it implies in the quality of her life. A feature common in depression is feeling angry and impatient with oneself, leading to low self-esteem. Recall that Suzanne felt she was a failure as a wife and mother as her illness progressed.

What would be reasonable goals for the problem of depression, considering Suzanne's situation at this time?

a. Acceptance of the limitations imposed by illness
b. Cheerful behavior
c. Improved self-esteem
d. Expression of feelings

c, d (Acceptance is usually attained later in the course of illness, but is sometimes not a goal that is acceptable to patients.)

### Frame 9

Which of these interventions are likely to be therapeutic?

a. Challenge her with more difficult self-care tasks.
b. Paint an optimistic picture of life on dialysis.
c. Encourage her to express her feelings by an interested and unhurried manner.
d. Show sympathy.
e. Set small, achievable goals.
f. Point out any improvement in her condition.
g. Treat her with respect.
h. Act cheerful with her.

c, e, f, g

## Frame 10

Match the nontherapeutic action with the way Suzanne could interpret it.

| Action | | Possible interpretation |
|---|---|---|
| 1. Paint an optimistic picture. | a. | Nonacceptance of her negative feelings |
| 2. Show sympathy. | b. | "You are pathetic." |
| 3. Challenge with more difficult tasks. | c. | "You can do more than you think, you're babying yourself." |
| 4. Act cheerful. | d. | "You are making mountains out of molehills." |

1. d or a
2. b
3. c
4. a or d

## Frame 11

What effect would these nontherapeutic interventions have on her self-esteem?

lower it even more

Again, timing becomes important. When Suzanne begins dialysis, she will feel better physically and her mental activity will improve. This may help in alleviating the depression.

As Ellen works with Suzanne, she will need to listen for Suzanne's viewpoint about her situation and for data related to the possible problems identified: fear, alteration in body image, and impairment of family and social relationships. If these become actual problems, Ellen will need to plan interventions.

## *Problem 5* — Alleviating Pain and Discomfort

## Frame 12

Recall that Suzanne complained of muscular cramps, aches, headaches, pruritus, discomforts from spending more time in bed, and painful procedures.

Select which goals would be realistic:

a. Decreased pruritus
b. No complaints of pain
c. Longer hours of uninterrupted sleep
d. Fewer complaints of pain

a, c, d

**Frame 13**

Choose the interventions which will decrease her pain and discomfort:

a. Use of bath oils and skin lotions
b. Warm packs for leg cramps
c. Use of antipruritic drugs
d. Teaching her methods to stop leg muscle cramps
e. Individually scheduled administration of analgesic drugs
f. Frequent change of position and back-rubs
g. All of the above

g

The skin care and comfort measures will also help to prevent skin breakdown.

Now a care plan has been developed to meet Suzanne's particular needs at this point in her illness. In Appendix B is a standard care plan for patients in end-stage renal failure.

Next you will study some general principles relative to dialysis, and then return to Suzanne and her experience with peritoneal dialysis.

**Frame 14**

Summary:

Chronic progressive renal disease involves a gradual loss of functioning nephrons due to inflammation and scarring of the glomerular membranes. The symptoms are progressive azotemia, proteinuria, hematuria, hypertension, fluid retention with edema, and physical signs of uremia in all body systems. It progresses in three phases:

1. Diminished renal reserve
2. Renal insufficiency
3. End-stage renal disease

Medical management involves: diet restriction of protein and sodium, diuretics, phosphorus-binding compounds, fluid restriction, antihypertensives, and correction of acidosis. Treatment of end-stage renal failure may be chronic dialysis or kidney transplantation.

See Appendix B for a sample nursing care plan.

# CHAPTER 12

## DIALYSIS: GENERAL INFORMATION

When medical management of acute or chronic renal failure is ineffective, dialysis is the next choice of treatment. This chapter defines dialysis, reviews important principles and the relationship to normal renal mechanisms, and discusses clinical indications for its use. When you complete this chapter, you will be able to

1. Define dialysis
2. Recognize that dialysate is similar in composition to serum by listing five electrolytes found in both
3. Identify the physical principles involved in solute removal or exchange and in fluid removal
4. Choose examples of the substances that are diffused in dialysis
5. Label a diagram showing the flow of solutes across the semipermeable membrane
6. Recognize the effect of dialysis on the renal mechanisms of protein homeostasis, reabsorption and excretion of solutes, fluid balance, and acid-base balance
7. Choose four clinical indications for dialysis.

### Chapter outline

Dialysis
- Definition
- Principles that make it work

Relationship to normal renal mechanisms
- Protein homeostasis
- Reabsorption and excretion of solutes
- Fluid balance
- Acid-base balance

Clinical indications for use
- Renal failure
- Other indications

# PART I DIALYSIS: DEFINITION AND PRINCIPLES

*Dialysis* refers to a diffusion and filtering process that occurs between solutions separated by a semipermeable membrane. This involves the removal of excess water, electrolytes, glucose, metabolic wastes, and dialyzable toxic materials from the body and the restoration of fluid, electrolyte and acid–base balance. This is accomplished by exposing blood to a special dialysis solution called dialysate.

*Panel 1*

Molecular Movement in Dialysis

*Blood*

*Semi-permeable membrane*

*Dialysate*

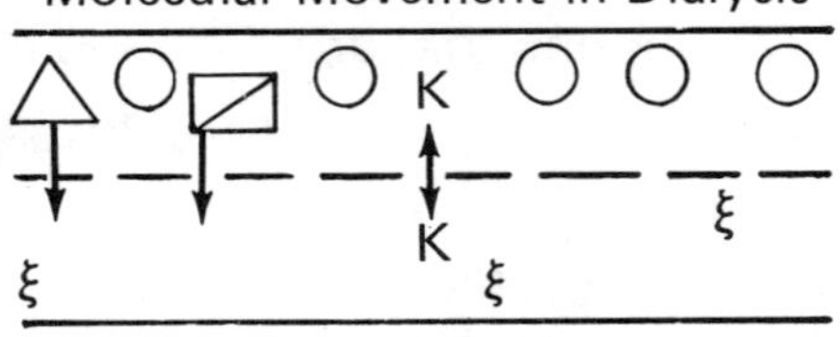


*Small molecules cross the membrane*

⧄ = *water*

K = *electrolytes, glucose*

Δ = *metabolic wastes, toxic materials*

*Large molecules will not cross the membrane*

○ = *red and white blood cells, protein, platelets*

ξ = *bacteria*

*Refer to Panel 1 for Frames 1, 2, and 3.*

## Frame 1

Dialysis is a diffusion and filtering process that occurs across a ____________ membrane and allows the exchange of (small/large) molecular substances.

semipermeable
small

## Frame 2

In dialysis the semipermeable membrane has microscopic pores which make it permeable to small molecules such as:

______________, | electrolytes (K, Na, and others)

______________, | water

______________, | metabolic wastes (urea, creatinine)

______________, and | glucose

______________. | toxic materials

## Frame 3

In dialysis the semipermeable membrane is relatively impermeable to large molecules such as:

______________, | red and white blood cells

______________, | platelets

______________, and | protein

______________. | bacteria

(The large molecules should *not* be exchanged during dialysis.)

## Frame 4

Define dialysis:

Dialysis is a process of diffusion and filtering that occurs between solutions separated by a semipermeable membrane and that allows the exchange of small molecular substances.

*Panel 2*

*Dialysate is the solution that determines the flow of water and solutes during dialysis.*

*This chart is a comparison of the electrolyte composition of dialysate and serum. To remove substances from the blood, the dialysate level is decreased or completely removed. To replace or restore a substance, the dialysate level is increased.*

| | *Serum Normals (mEq/liter)* | *Peritoneal dialysate (mEq/liter)* | *Hemo-dialysate (mEq/liter)* |
|---|---|---|---|
| *Sodium* | *135–145* | *140–141* | *135* |
| *Chloride* | *98–102* | *101–102* | *100.5* |
| *Potassium* | *3.5–5.5* | *0–4* | *0–4* |
| *Calcium* | *4.25–5* | *3.5–4* | *3* |
| *Magnesium* | *1.5–2.5* | *1.0–1.5* | *1* |

## Frame 5

Refer to Panel 2. Are the electrolyte components of dialysate (similar to/different from) the components of normal serum?

similar to

## Frame 6

In the blood, about 40% of the calcium ions are bound to protein molecules. Therefore, only 60% of the total serum calcium is available to cross a semipermeable membrane. To keep a balance between the dialysate and serum calcium levels, the dialysate level is about 60% of the serum level, in both hemodialysate and peritoneal dialysate.

Refer to Panel 2

1. If the normal serum calcium level is 5 mEq/liter, how many mEq of calcium would be added to dialysate to equal the 60% of unbound calcium?

1. $0.60 \times 5 = 3$ mEq/liter

2. Is this approximately the calcium level of both hemodialysate and peritoneal dialysate?

2. Yes, peritoneal = 3.5–4 mEq/liter, hemodialysate = 3 mEq/liter

3. About 40% of serum calcium is bound to ____________, making it (available/unavailable) to cross a semipermeable membrane.

3. protein unavailable

## Frame 7

Dialysis must also help correct acid–base balance by restoring serum bicarbonate. Bicarbonate added directly to dialysate would combine with the calcium and magnesium and form a chalklike precipitate. Instead, precursors of bicarbonate such as lactate or acetate are in dialysate. (Precursors are chemicals that can be changed into the desired substance.) They diffuse into the blood and are metabolized to bicarbonate by the liver.

| Serum | Peritoneal dialysate | Hemo-dialysate |
|---|---|---|
| Bicarbonate = 26–28 mEq/liter | Lactate = 43–45 mEq/liter | Acetate = 35 mEq/liter |

1. The level of lactate or acetate in the dialysate is (higher/lower) than in serum.

1. higher

2. Therefore, the acetate or lactate will diffuse (into/out of) the patient's blood.

2. into

3. When the lactate or acetate is in the patient's blood, it is used to (increase/decrease) the patient's supply of base–bicarbonate.

3. increase

Recent studies have revealed patients who are unable to convert the acetate into bicarbonate. Researchers are developing ways to mix bicarbonate-containing dialysate.

## Frame 8

Glucose is another component in dialysate. About 200 mg/100 ml may be added routinely to hemodialysate to prevent hypoglycemia and to prevent protein stores being used for energy. Glucose in the form of dextrose is the component of peritoneal dialysate that determines how much fluid will be removed by an osmotic gradient (1.5–4.25 g/liter). Occasionally, an osmotic gradient may also be needed to remove fluid during hemodialysis.

To remove more fluid by osmosis during dialysis, the concentration of dextrose would need to be (increased/decreased).

increased

## Frame 9

Refer to Panel 2.

Mrs. Rice is one of the dialysis patients.

Her laboratory report showed

K = 6.2 mEq/liter

Na = 131 mEq/liter

Mg = 3 mEq/liter

1. Indicate with an arrow whether her serum levels are higher or lower than the dialysate level.
2. Choose the correct element(s):
   Since dialysis will correct Mrs. Rice's electrolyte imbalances, the excess (K, Na, Mg) will be removed, and depleted (K, Na, Mg) will be replaced.

1.
   K ↑
   Na ↓
   Mg ↑
2. excess K, Mg
   depleted Na

## Frame 10

List five electrolytes found in dialysate:

Potassium, sodium, calcium, magnesium, chloride

## Frame 11

*Diffusion* is one of three physical processes utilized in dialysis. Elevated serum solutes are removed by decreasing the level in dialysate and low serum solutes are replaced by increasing the dialysate level.

Indicate by an arrow (⟶/⟵) the direction of diffusion of the following solutes.

1.

| Dialysate | Blood |
|---|---|
| Urea | Urea<br>••••<br>•••• |

2.

| Dialysate | Blood |
|---|---|
| Potassium<br>•••• | Potassium<br>••••<br>•••<br>• |

3.

| Dialysate | Blood |
|---|---|
| Calcium<br>••• | Calcium<br>••••• |

(Hint: see Frame 6.)

4.

| Dialysate | Blood |
|---|---|
| Potassium<br>•••• | Potassium<br>••• |

5.

| Dialysate | Blood |
|---|---|
| Acetate<br>••<br>•••<br>••• | |

(Hint: see Frame 7.)

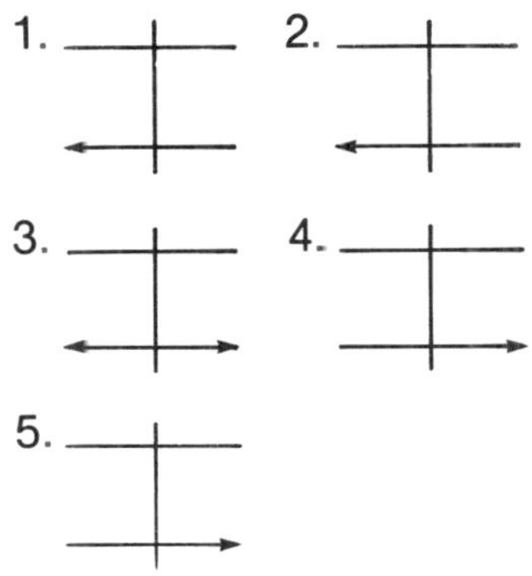


## Frame 12

In the diagram below, indicate with an arrow the direction of solute exchange.

| Blood | | Dialysate | |
|---|---|---|---|
| Potassium | 7 mEq/liter | Potassium | 2 mEq/liter |
| Magnesium | 3 mEq/liter | Magnesium | 1.5 mEq/liter |
| Calcium | 5 mEq/liter | Calcium | 3 mEq/liter |
| Urea | 90 mg/100 ml | Urea | 0 |
| Creatinine | 14 mg/100 ml | Creatinine | 0 |
| Glucose | 165 mg/100 ml | Glucose | 200 mg/100 ml |
| Bicarbonate | 24 mEq/liter | Acetate | 35 mEq/liter |

(Hint: see Frame 7.)

Potassium ⟶

Magnesium ⟶

Calcium—no exchange (Forty percent of serum calcium is protein bound.)

Urea ⟶

Creatinine ⟶

Glucose ⟵

Bicarbonate ⟵

### Frame 13

Solute removal or replacement in dialysis is accomplished by the process of ____________.

diffusion

### Frame 14

1. Osmosis is the transfer of ____________ to an area of higher concentration of solutes.

   It is a second process used in dialysis.
2. Glucose is added to dialysate to ____________ osmosis.

1. water
2. increase

### Frame 15

The third process utilized in dialysis is *filtration* of fluid due to positive or negative pressure gradients. Gravity is a positive pressure, suction is a negative pressure. Filtration will be discussed in Chapter 15.

# PART II RELATIONSHIP TO NORMAL RENAL MECHANISMS

## Frame 16

*Protein Homeostasis*

The patient being maintained on dialysis can usually resume an unrestricted protein diet as the metabolic wastes are removed during dialysis. This promotes protein homeostasis and fosters the building up of cells.

1. What is this building up process called?
2. Why can the dialysis diet be more liberal in protein intake than a renal failure diet?

1. anabolism
2. Dialysis will remove the metabolic wastes.

## Frame 17

*Reabsorption and excretion of solutes*

When the kidneys are damaged, the renal mechanism of solute excretion and reabsorption is carried out by dialysis. Which of these statements are true?

1. ______ Dialysis removes accumulated by-products of protein metabolism.
2. ______ Dialysis readjusts the level of body electrolytes.
3. ______ Dialysis removes toxic substances.

1. True
2. True
3. True

## Frame 18

*Fluid balance*

True or false:

______ Body fluid balance is readjusted because dialysis removes excess fluid.

True

## Frame 19

*Acid–base balance*

1. Lactate or acetate in dialysate diffuses into the blood and is converted to what substance?
2. Does this increase or decrease the body's alkali reserve?
3. What involvement does the liver have in this process? (Refer to Frame 7 if you can't remember.)

1. Bicarbonate
2. Increase
3. The liver converts the lactate or acetate to bicarbonate.

# PART III CLINICAL INDICATIONS FOR USE

## Frame 20

Dialysis is commonly used to treat acute and chronic renal failure. It may also be used in cases of intoxication with a lethal dose of a dialyzable drug or poison. Drugs such as barbiturates, meprobamate and glutethimide (Doriden) and metals like lead and arsenic, are dialyzable.

Dialysis is being used to remove various toxins or other substances from the blood that are thought to be related to diseases such as schizophrenia, oxalosis and chronic hyperuricemia.

Dialysis can be used to remove fluid retained in cases of congestive heart failure and pulmonary edema that have not responded to diuretics. Occasionally, electrolyte imbalances such as acidosis, hyperkalemia, hyperuricemia, or hyponatremia may be corrected by dialysis.

From the following diagnoses, choose the ones for which dialysis is indicated:

a. Snowmobile accident with crush injuries and acute renal failure
b. Renal failure secondary to chronic glomerulonephritis
c. Congestive heart failure responding to diuretics
d. Lethal overdose of meprobamate
e. Intractable pulmonary edema

a, b, d, e

## Frame 21

Summary:

Dialysis is a process of diffusion and filtration or osmosis across a semipermeable membrane. Body levels of small molecular substances, normally removed or restored by the kidney, are corrected during dialysis.

The composition of a special solution called dialysate determines the flow of water and solutes across the semipermeable membrane. Dialysate is similar in composition to normal serum.

Dialysis promotes protein homeostasis and corrects solute, fluid, and acid-base balances in the body.

Indications for dialysis include acute renal failure, chronic renal failure, intractable edema or electrolyte imbalances, and intoxication with a lethal dose of a dialyzable drug or poison.

# CHAPTER 13
## PERITONEAL DIALYSIS

Peritoneal dialysis has become a simple and readily available method of dialysis. Its successful outcome depends on intelligent, well-organized nursing care. After completing this chapter, you will be able to

1. Identify selected features of the peritoneal membrane relative to dialysis
2. List the physical principles involved in peritoneal dialysis
3. Predict how varying types of dialyzing fluid affect exchange
4. List the nursing actions necessary to prepare a patient for peritoneal dialysis
5. Describe the procedure for insertion of the catheter and infusion of fluid
6. Develop a nursing care plan for a patient on peritoneal dialysis.

### Chapter outline

- Principles
  - The peritoneum as a dialyzing membrane
  - The effect of osmosis
  - The effect of diffusion and filtration
- Procedure
  - Insertion of the catheter
  - Dialysate infusion
  - Drainage of dialysate
- Patient Care During Dialysis
  - Intake and output records
  - Complications
    - Physical
    - Technical
- Nursing Care Plan
  - Nursing observations
  - Nursing interventions during dialysis
  - Assisting the patient to cope with treatment

# PART I
# PRINCIPLES

In peritoneal dialysis, a solution is infused into the abdominal cavity through a closed drainage system. It uses the peritoneum as a dialyzing membrane to replace kidney function. The peritoneum is the membrane that forms a sac as it lines the abdominal cavity and surrounds the abdominal organs. The surface area of the peritoneum is about the same as that of all the glomerular membranes, about 22,000 cm². This provides a large surface for dialysis.

## Frame 1

Here is a diagram of the peritoneum, represented by the heavy white line.

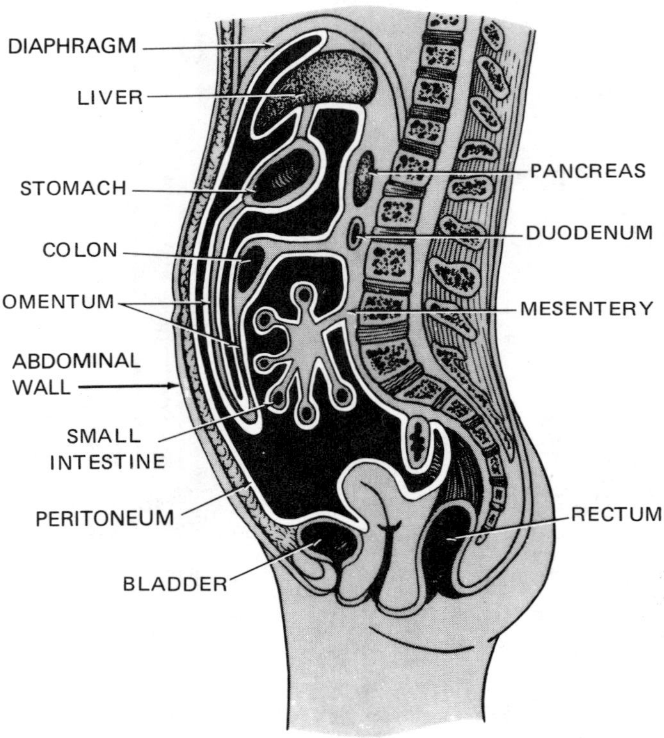


Figure 46

True or false:

1. ______ Peritoneum lines the abdominal wall.

1. True

2. ______ There is a layer of peritoneum around all the organs that lie in the abdomen.

2. True

3. ______ The abdominal cavity really has a big empty space as is shown in the diagram.

3. False (It has a *potential* space.)

4. ______ If fluid were instilled in the abdominal cavity it would flow around the organs, and space would be created through abdominal distention.

4. True

5. ______ A layer of the peritoneum lies right under the diaphragm.

5. True

6. ______ Abdominal distention due to fluid instillation would have no effect upon respiratory adequacy.

6. False (It would cause pressure on the diaphragm.)

## Frame 2

Now look more closely at the peritoneum. This figure shows one loop of bowel and mesentery. Note that the peritoneum is right next to the rich capillary network in the intestinal walls and mesentery. Dialysate is instilled through a catheter into the peritoneal space, bathing the intestinal loops.

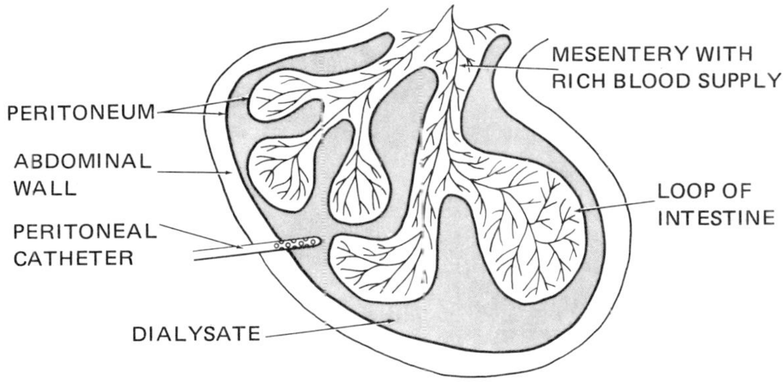


Figure 47

The exchange of water and electrolytes in peritoneal dialysis would take place between these fluids: ______________, flowing through capillaries in the abdominal, mesenteric and intestinal walls, and ______________ infused into the abdominal cavity.

blood, dialysate

## Frame 3

By a combination of osmosis, diffusion, and filtration, excess fluid and electrolytes are balanced. The peritoneal membrane is permeable to small molecules of electrolytes and water, but is less permeable to large molecules of protein and dextrose.

Therefore, dialysate solutions have a basic electrolyte composition similar to plasma; and dextrose is added in varying amounts to increase tonicity (or osmotic pressure).

1. If the dialysate solution was hypertonic, osmosis would cause water to move in which of these directions? — 1. a
   a. Blood to dialysate
   b. Dialysate to blood
2. Which of these dialysate solutions would draw the most water from the blood? — 2. b
   a. 1.5% dextrose
   b. 4.25% dextrose
3. As the dextrose solution pulls the water through the membrane, the other solutes in the blood also cross with the water. This is sometimes called "osmotic drag."

   Increasing the dextrose content of the solution, therefore, increases the removal of urea from the blood. Why would this happen? — 3. b
   a. Urea is electromagnetically attracted to glucose.
   b. A high osmotic pressure will pull more solutes out along with the water.
   c. Urea is a large molecule.
4. If the dialysate had a lower concentration of potassium than the serum potassium level, which of these ways would potassium diffuse? — 4. a
   a. From blood to dialysate
   b. From dialysate to blood
   c. No movement

The third process which aids peritoneal dialysis is filtration. This is hydrostatic pressure which pushes fluids through the capillary and peritoneal membranes, into the dialysate. Gravity also forces the fluid to drain out of the abdomen into a bottle at a lower level.

## Frame 4

If the dialyzing fluid is left in the abdominal cavity too long, the blood and dialysate begin to reach equilibrium. Sugar molecules begin to be absorbed, despite their size. This reduces the osmotic pressure of the dialysate and decreases the removal of water and urea. This is why dialysate is left in the abdominal cavity 20 minutes or less, and then is drained out into a collection bottle. The period that dialysate is left in the abdomen is called dwell time or dialysis time.

1. True or false:
   a. ______ The osmotic pressure of dialysate is due mostly to dextrose concentration.
   b. ______ Urea is removed along with water by osmotic drag.
   c. ______ Prolonged contact between dialysate and blood increases effectiveness of dialysate.
2. Choose the dialysis that would remove the most water and solutes:
   a. Three exchanges with 1-hour dwell times
   b. Ten exchanges with 20-minute dwell times

1.
   a. True
   b. True
   c. False
2. b

## Frame 5

Summary:

In peritoneal dialysis

The peritoneum is the dialyzing membrane that allows passage of water and small molecules of electrolyte and waste products. It is less permeable to sugar molecules.

The dialysate is similar to plasma in electrolyte concentration, and tonicity is regulated by adding various amounts of dextrose. Dialysate comes in contact with capillaries as it is infused into the abdominal cavity.

Osmosis, diffusion, and filtration are the forces behind the removal of excess water and metabolic wastes and the equilibration of electrolytes. This process is accomplished using multiple infusions of dialysate with dwell times of about 20 minutes.

# PART II PROCEDURE

Now you will learn about the experience Suzanne Rice had while on peritoneal dialysis. When you left her in Chapter 11, she was suffering from severe uremic symptoms. Her chief nursing problems were fluid and electrolyte imbalances, acidosis, negative protein balance, mental cloudiness, depression, pain and discomfort, and lack of strength and mobility.

Suzanne had an access site for hemodialysis (a fistula) surgically created in her arm. However, it was not ready for use. In addition, her physicians thought that she should begin on peritoneal dialysis to avoid the risk of seizures from a more rapid shift of fluid and electrolytes during hemodialysis.

The first step in peritoneal dialysis is the insertion of the catheter. This can be done on a temporary basis, using much the same procedure as for abdominal paracentesis, in which a Silastic or Teflon catheter is introduced through a trocar or with a stylet. (See Panel 1.)

## *PANEL 1*

*HOW THE CATHETER IS INSERTED*

*Before the doctor arrives, gather the following equipment: disposable razor and blade, dialysis administration set, peritoneal dialysis solution (as ordered), local anesthesia (Xylocaine 1%), sterile gloves, Betadine solution and ointment, suture and needle #2-0 silk, and Elastoplast. Also get a sterile prepackaged dialysis tray with catheter, connector, syringes, needles, sterile dressings, and fine mesh gauze.*

*Explain the procedure to the patient and get his signed consent. Weigh him to obtain a baseline weight, and take temperature, pulse, respiration, and blood pressure readings. Have him empty his bladder to reduce the risk of bladder perforation during insertion. Make him comfortable in a supine position, and shave his abdomen from umbilicus to 5 cm below it. The doctor will then begin the insertion procedure.*

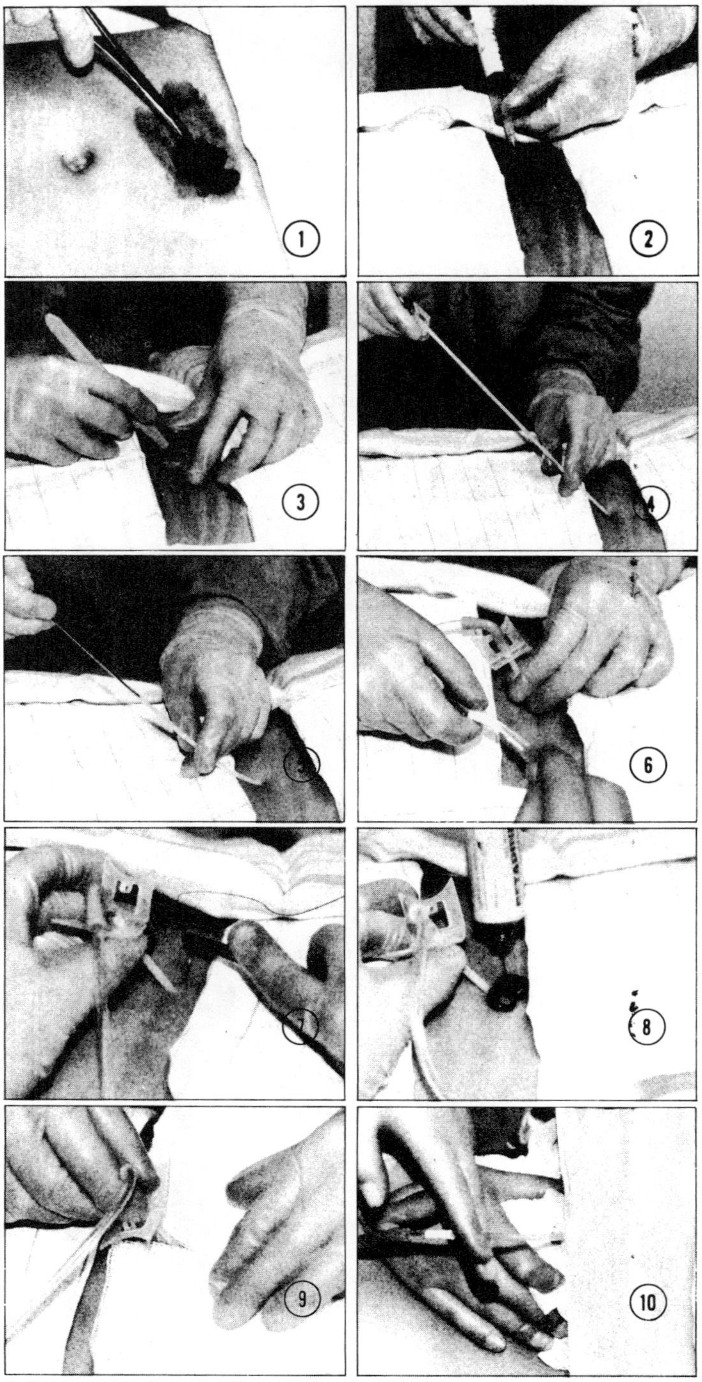

1. *First, he swabs the skin with Betadine, to eliminate surface bacteria.*
2. *After draping the patient, he then infiltrates the skin and subcutaneous tissues with a local anesthetic.*
3. *He makes a small midline stab wound 3 to 5 cm below the umbilicus.*
4. *Next, he inserts the peritoneal catheter with stylet through the incision. If the patient is thin, he may inject 1 to 2 liters of fluid through the incision before inserting the stylet. This allows free movement of the mesentery and bowel when the stylet perforates the peritoneum.*
5. *With the stylet in place, the patient raises his head to tighten his abdominal muscles. This makes penetration easier and reduces the risk of injury to the intra-abdominal organs. When the doctor punctures the peritoneum, he will hear an audible pop and feel markedly less resistance. He then removes the stylet.*
6. *He maneuvers the catheter into place and connects it to the administration set and dialyzing solution.*
7. *With purse-string suture, he then closes the skin looping the suture around the catheter and tying it in place.*
8. *He applies Betadine ointment or another antibacterial agent to the incision site.*
9. *Then, he places a sterile dressing around the catheter.*
10. *After padding the area with more sterile gauze, he applies Elastoplast tape to keep the dressing and catheter in place. He is then ready to allow 2 liters of warmed 37°C. dialyzing solution to run in rapidly, over a period of 10 minutes.*

P. Dolan and H. Greene, "Renal Failure and Peritoneal Dialysis," *Nursing 75*, 5:7 (1975) p. 48.

Long-term access to the abdominal cavity was gained for Suzanne by surgically implanting the catheter through a tunnel of subcutaneous tissue and then into the peritoneum. This figure shows one kind of peritoneal catheter in place. The Dacron felt cuffs prevent movement of the catheter, bowel herniation, and infection. Tissue begins to grow around and through the felt, which helps to seal the tunnel. The connector and disposable rubber closure cap facilitate repeated sterile connection to the administration set.

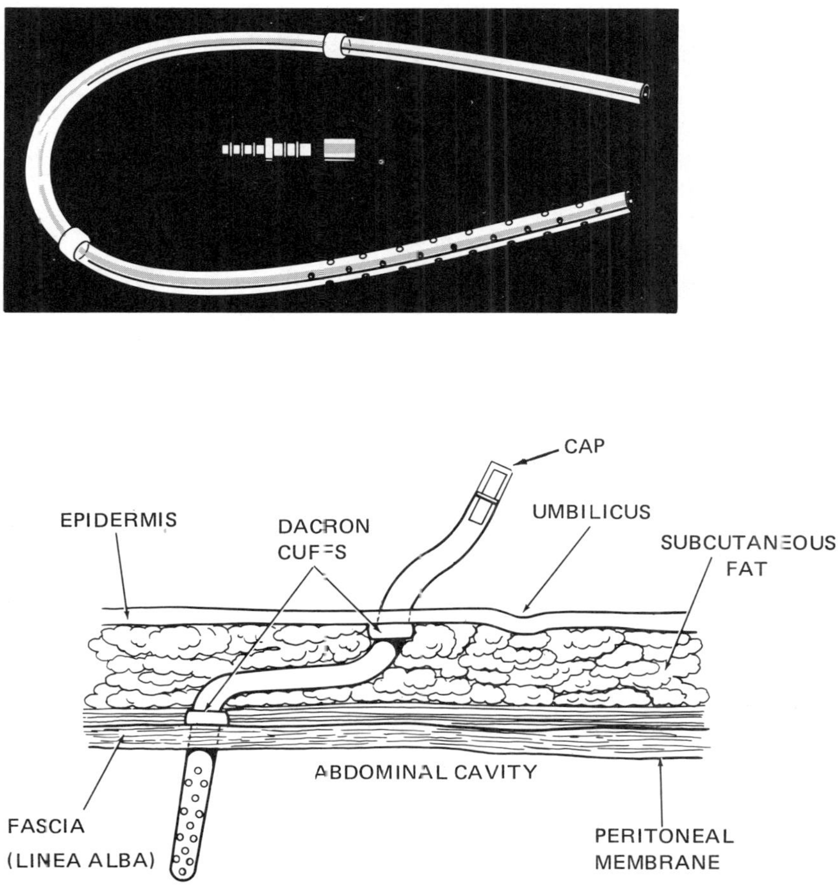


Figure 48

## Frame 6

Refer to Panel 1.

1. Why is it important that the patient void before insertion of the peritoneal catheter?

   a. For intake and output records
   b. A full bladder could be punctured as the peritoneal catheter is placed.
   c. To prevent patient restlessness during procedure

   *Answer:* 1. b (See the figure in Frame 1 for anatomic relationships.)

2. List the data that needs to be documented on the chart before beginning dialysis:

   _______________
   _______________
   _______________
   _______________
   _______________

   *Answer:* 2. Weight, temperature, blood pressure, pulse, respirations

3. What is the usual site for insertion of the peritoneal catheter?

   *Answer:* 3. 3–5 cm below the umbilicus

During insertion of the peritoneal catheter, the nurse, Ellen, warmed the dialysate to body temperature by placing the bottle in a water bath. Warming the solution enhances the urea clearance by 35%, decreases the patient's discomfort, and prevents loss of the patient's body heat.

Then, Ellen hung the bottle of dialysate, let it flow rapidly into Suzanne's abdominal cavity (5–10 min) and allowed a 20-minute dwell time. She then drained the solution, which took 5–10 minutes. This cycle was repeated for the prescribed number of hours.

There are various kinds of administration sets, which are designed on the same principle as IV administration equipment. Automated peritoneal dialysis systems are also available. These are like hemodialysis machines in that they deliver a warmed dialysate which can be diluted from a concentrated solution through a closed sterile circuit. They have built-in monitors, and they automatically cycle infusion and drainage of the dialysate at a more rapid rate.

## Frame 7

Peritoneal dialysis is done in cycles or exchanges:

Phase 1 Infusion or inflow: 10 min
Phase 2 Dwell time: 20 min
Phase 3 Drainage: 10–30 min

The length of each phase may vary depending on the treatment routines established and specific needs of patients

Match each phase with the effect taking place:

1. ____________ Dialysate in peritoneal cavity is exchanging water, wastes, and electrolytes with blood in adjacent vessels. — Phase 2
2. ____________ Dialysate flows out of the peritoneal cavity by gravity, removing waste products. — Phase 3
3. ____________ Dialysate flows into the abdominal cavity by gravity. — Phase 1

## Frame 8

Before beginning dialysis, Ellen warmed the dialysate in a pan of water to 37°C. Select the reason(s) why she did this? — a, b

a. Warm temperatures cause vasodilation and would bring more blood to the area for exchange.
b. Cold dialysate could cause chills and heat loss.
c. Another example of nursing ritual.

## Frame 9

Warming the dialysate is one factor that affects the rate at which solutes exchange. Which of the following would also affect the rate of exchange?

a. The large peritoneal membrane surface (22,000 cm$^2$)
b. The concentration gradient
c. A large peritoneal catheter
d. The duration of dialysate and peritoneum contact

a (This provides almost the same surface area as the kidney.)

b (Diffusion depends on the concentration gradient.)

d (After about 20 min equilibration is reached and the concentration gradient is no longer effective.)

## Frame 10

Infection is probably the greatest risk involved in peritoneal dialysis. From the following list, choose situations which could result in infection:

a. Use of sterile technique to swab bottle tops with antiseptic
b. Drips from the water bath running down the bottle and catheter
c. Use of the bathroom sink to warm the bottles
d. Introduction of bacteria when medications are added
e. Sterile technique in handling tubing and connectors

b, c, d

## Frame 11

Summary:

A peritoneal catheter is inserted 3-5 cm below the umbilicus, under sterile conditions. Preparation of the patient includes: signed consent, void before procedure, record weight, temperature, pulse, respiration, and blood pressure.

The dialysate is warmed to body temperature and instilled in this routine:

Phase 1 Infusion: 10 min
Phase 2 Dwell time: 20 min
Phase 3 Drainage time: 10–30 min

# PART III PATIENT CARE DURING DIALYSIS

Here are the medical orders written for Mrs. Rice:

*Routine Peritoneal Dialysis Orders*

1. *Informed, written consent signed.*
2. *Weigh patient prior to the procedure and every A.M. with empty abdomen.*
3. *Accurate dialysis fluid record.*
4. *BP, P and R $\bar{q}$* 2 Hrs. *Notify physician if b.p. is* > 160/94 *or* < 90/60.
5. *Temperature $\bar{q}$* 4 Hrs. *If temp.* > 101°, *notify physician.*
6. *CVP if ordered.*
7. *Run dialysis on* 1 *hour cycle as follows:*
   *Run in two (2) liters of fluid rapidly (IV standard extended to full height with clamp wide open.) Clamp tube for* 20 *minutes and then drain for rest of cycle.*
8. *Use fluids on following schedule:*
   *Start with two (2) liters of Dianeal® 1.5% Dextrose. If returns from previous cycle are:*
   *A. less than* 1800 *ml, use two (2) liters of Dianeal® with 4.25% Dextrose.*
   *B. over* 2000 *ml, use two (2) liters of Dianeal® 1.5% Dextrose.*
9. *To each run add: (one only of the two liters)*
   50 *units of Heparin*
   4 *mEq KCl.*
   — *mg. 1% Xylocaine*
10. *Maintain on dialysis for 36 hours.*

Suzanne was begun on hourly cycles as ordered. Heparin is added to the dialysate to keep the catheter from plugging with blood clots or fibrin. The level of potassium (0–4 mEq/liter) is determined by the patient's serum $K^+$. After hyperkalemia is corrected, the dialysate amount will be enough to maintain a normal serum $K^+$ and prevent hypokalemia. Xylocaine may be used to decrease the discomfort. During the first few cycles, Mrs. Rice complained of a feeling of fullness. During the eighth exchange, the drainage became less than 1,800 ml, so Ellen used the more concentrated dialysate for the next cycle. This time the results were better, with 2,500 ml of drainage recovered.

## Recording Intake and Output

### Frame 12

One of the most important features of nursing care is the exact recording of intake and output.

If fluid is retained by the patient this is noted as a + amount.

If you get back more fluid than you infuse, this is recorded as a - amount.

Then at the end of the exchange, the patient's gain or loss can be calculated.

Example: (See chart that follows.)

During the first exchange, Suzanne was given 2,000 ml, and there was 2,100 ml of drainage. This means she lost 100 ml, so it is recorded as -100.

During the next exchange, 1,950 ml was infused and 1,850 ml was returned. This means that she retained 100 ml, so it is recorded + 100.

On the third exchange, 1,900 ml was infused and 2,050 ml returned. She then lost 150 ml, recorded as -150.

The difference between inflow and outflow is calculated and compared with any gains or losses in the previous exchange. The present status is then calculated and recorded.

Problems: Continue this recording on the chart:

| *Time* | *Exchange #* | *Volume In* | *Volume Out* |
|---|---|---|---|
| 4:30 | 4 | 2,050 | 1,900 |
| 5:30 | 5 | 2,000 | 2,150 |
| 6:30 | 6 | 2,050 | 2,200 |

| *Time* | *Exchange #* | *Volume In* | *Volume Out* | *Fluid balance* | *Previous* | *Present* |
|---|---|---|---|---|---|---|
| 1:45 | 1 | 2,000 | 2,100 | -100 | | |
| 2:30 | 2 | 1,950 | 1,850 | + 100 | -100 | 0 |
| 3:30 | 3 | 1,900 | 2,050 | -150 | 0 | -150 |
| | | | | | | |
| | | | | | | |
| | | | | | | |

| *Time* | *Exchange #* | *Volume In* | *Volume Out* | *Fluid balance* | *Previous* | *Present* |
|---|---|---|---|---|---|---|
| 4:30 | 4 | 2,050 | 1,900 | + 150 | -150 | 0 |
| 5:30 | 5 | 2,000 | 2,150 | -150 | 0 | -150 |
| 6:30 | 6 | 2,050 | 2,200 | -150 | -150 | -300 |

The procedure for recording intake and output during dialysis may differ between hospitals. The important thing is that all nurses are consistent, so that recording is accurate.

## Frame 13

Recording of accurately measured dialysate intake and drainage is of utmost importance in following the patient's fluid status. The exact number of ml's in each bottle of dialysate should be recorded.

Mark these statements true or false:

1. ______ Flushing air from the tubing may decrease the number of ml's.
2. ______ Adding medications will increase the volume of dialysate.
3. ______ Each liter bottle comes from the manufacturer with exactly 1,000 ml.

1. True
2. True
3. False. (Manufacturers usually have an excess of 50 ml or more in each bottle. An extra 50 ml each cycle can quickly throw off the recorded fluid balance.)

## Complications: Physical

### Frame 14

Hypotension and shock may occur if too much fluid is removed, especially when a hypertonic solution is used. Ellen would need to be alert for which of these symptoms?

a. Edema
b. Rapid weight loss
c. Rapid pulse
d. Persistent drop in blood pressure

b, c, d

### Frame 15

Fluid overload can occur if the patient retains fluid from the dialysate. Which of these symptoms would be present?

a. Hypertension
b. Dyspnea
c. Chest pain
d. Weight loss

a, b, c

Solutes can also become unbalanced during dialysis. If the dwell time is prolonged, dextrose could be absorbed, causing hyperglycemia. Electrolytes such as sodium and potassium are also susceptible to imbalance.

### Frame 16

One of the most important considerations is respiratory care. The patient's full abdomen puts pressure on the diaphragm. Hypoventilation is also associated with bed rest and abdominal discomfort, and these factors make the patient susceptible to pneumonia.

Choose the intervention(s) which would be helpful to respiratory care:

a. Turning from side to side
b. Leg exercises
c. Deep breathing, coughing
d. None of the above

a, c (Leg exercises prevent venous stasis, but are not related to respiratory care.)

If the patient becomes dyspneic during dialysis, drain the dialysate and call the physician.

Abdominal pain is a common problem during dialysis, and severity depends on the individual. This is probably caused by the abdominal distention, chemical irritation of the peritoneum, or incomplete drainage of solution.

Severe pain after the first 24 hours may indicate peritonitis or paralytic ileus.

During the 28th exchange, Mrs. Rice complained of severe pain, especially during inflow. This became worse during the next exchange and the dialysate drainage was cloudy. Her temperature had gone up suddenly to 101.6°F. Ellen sent a sample of fluid to the lab for a culture, and antibiotics were ordered both IV and in the dialysate solution. During the acute stage of peritonitis, Suzanne felt very ill with chills, nausea, cramping, abdominal pain, and temperature over 103°F.

Because of the peritonitis, she remained on continuous dialysis for 72 hours, as antibiotics could be constantly instilled. This treatment was successful, the peritonitis subsided, and Suzanne was switched to a daily 12-hour dialysis for 5 days.

## Frame 17

Dialysate drainage is normally clear and straw colored. (Right after insertion of the peritoneal catheter, the first few outflows may show slight bleeding due to the procedure.) Match the abnormal appearance of dialysate with one possible cause.

| | | | | Answers |
|---|---|---|---|---|
| 1. ______ | Bloody | a. | Infection | 1. c |
| | | b. | Bowel perforation | |
| 2. ______ | Cloudy | c. | Intraabdominal bleeding | 2. a |
| 3. ______ | Fecal | d. | Bladder perforation | 3. b |

Severe diarrhea during or after the first exchange may also indicate bowel perforation. The sudden production of urine and need to void may indicate bladder perforation. The exchange should be stopped, and the physician notified.

## Complications: Technical

Incomplete recovery of fluid with each exchange

The fluid removed should be at least equal to the inflow amount. If the catheter tip is caught in folds of omentum, or if the catheter is clogged, less fluid may drain. The heparin which was ordered for Suzanne should prevent clotting or fibrin deposits. Drainage can be facilitated by

Turning the patient from side to side

Elevating the head of the bed

Gently massaging the abdomen.

Persistent bleeding or leaking from around the catheter

Wet dressings around the catheter are a source of bacterial contamination, so frequent dressing changes and use of sterile plastic drapes are indicated.

Accidental catheter displacement

The physician will probably place a purse string suture around the catheter to prevent this problem.

### Frame 18

Summary:

Intake and output are recorded accurately, and the amount of fluid gained or lost by the patient is calculated after each exchange.

Physical complications include: hypotension and hypovolemia, fluid overload, hypostatic pneumonia, infection, perforation of bowel or bladder, and intraabdominal bleeding.

Technical complications include: incomplete recovery of fluid with each exchange and persistent bleeding or leakage around the catheter.

# PART IV NURSING CARE PLAN

## Nursing Care Plan

Since the dialysis was taking over some of the kidney functions Suzanne had lost, she no longer had abnormal amounts of urea, creatinine, and other waste products in her blood. Body fluids were balanced, her blood pressure came down, and electrolyte balance was restored.

One problem that still remained was protein imbalance. The peritoneum is permeable to many protein molecules, so protein loss is unavoidable during peritoneal dialysis. The physicians monitored Suzanne's serum albumin level, and ordered IV infusions of albumin when needed. Her diet was also high in essential protein to help replace the losses. Her diet was still restricted in sodium and potassium, and she was to keep her fluid intake under 500 ml/day.

## Nursing Observations: Monitor effectiveness of dialysis and adequacy of nursing care

*Problem 1*

Use the Response Indicator to develop a list of observations that should be made to judge fluid balance status during dialysis.
Squares numbered: ____________

*Problem 2*

Now choose the observations that directly measure waste clearance and solute exchange during dialysis. Squares numbered: ____________

*Problem 3*

Decide which observations will pick up frequently occurring secondary complications during dialysis. (Do not include fluid balance again.) Squares numbered: ____________

| Response Indicator | | | | |
|---|---|---|---|---|
| Fluid intake and output 1 | Character of drainage returns 2 | Neurologic checks 3 | Blood pressure (and CVP if ordered) 4 | Breath sounds 5 |
| Serum albumin 6 | Serum electrolytes 7 | Temperature 8 | Pulse 9 | Respirations 10 |
| BUN and serum creatinine 11 | Blood sugar levels 12 | Pressure areas on skin over bony prominences 13 | ECG monitoring 14 | Weight 15 |

| Response Indicator | | | | |
|---|---|---|---|---|
| Fluid intake and output 1 | Character of drainage returns 2 | Neurologic checks 3 | Blood pressure (and CVP if ordered) 4 | Breath sounds 5 |
| Serum albumin 6 | Serum electrolytes 7 | Temperature 8 | Pulse 9 | Respirations 10 |
| BUN and serum creatinine 11 | Blood sugar levels 12 | Pressure areas on skin over bony prominences 13 | ECG monitoring 14 | Weight 15 |

## Comments

*Problem 1* — Fluid Balance

Suggested responses: 1, 4, 9, and 15

O 1, 4, 9, 15

The best indicator of fluid status is the accurate recording of fluid intake (dialysis inflow and oral intake) and output (dialysis drainage, urine, feces, emesis). Blood pressure and pulse will change if there is a significant gain or serious loss of fluid. To review these patterns, see Frames 14 and 15. The weight should be compared to the predialysis weight.

I 5, 10, 14

If you included respirations and breath sounds because these will change in fluid overload, you were correct in your thinking. ECG monitoring could give data showing left ventricular strain in fluid overload states, but this type of monitoring is not routine for patients on peritoneal dialysis who do not have concurrent cardiac problems.

*Problem 2* — Waste Clearance and Solute Exchange

Suggested responses: 6, 7, 11, and 12.

O 6, 7, 11, 12

Clearance of waste products from the blood is reflected in the BUN and serum creatinine. Loss of protein from the serum into the dialysate is monitored by the serum albumin levels. If dwell times are too long, dextrose from the dialysate can cross the peritoneum and raise blood levels.

I 3, 9, 14

You are correct if you have included neurologic checks because metabolic imbalances (such as a high BUN) may affect the level of consciousness. Also, potassium imbalances causing arrhythmias might be detected in the pulse or ECG monitoring.

*Problem 3* — Secondary Complications

Suggested responses: 2, 5, 6, 8, 10, 12, and 13

O 2

The appearance of drainage can indicate infection, bleeding or bowel perforation. Cloudy drainage, pain, and elevated temperature are the signs of infection.

| Response Indicator | | | | |
|---|---|---|---|---|
| Fluid intake and output 1 | Character of drainage returns 2 | Neurologic checks 3 | Blood pressure (and CVP if ordered) 4 | Breath sounds 5 |
| Serum albumin 6 | Serum electrolytes 7 | Temperature 8 | Pulse 9 | Respirations 10 |
| BUN and serum creatinine 11 | Blood sugar levels 12 | Pressure areas on skin over bony prominences 13 | ECG monitoring 14 | Weight 15 |

O 5, 8, 10

These observations: elevated temperature, fast respirations (also dyspnea, cyanosis, chest pain) and abnormal breath sounds (rales, rhonchi, absence of sounds) indicate hypostatic pneumonia. You may wish to review Frame 16 for more information.

O 6, 12

Continuous loss of protein, as reflected by low serum albumin levels, can lead to negative protein balance with lack of protein to rebuild cells and enzymes, and decreased plasma osmolality.

If sugar from the dialysate is absorbed, hyperglycemia may occur. This observation is particularly important if the patient is diabetic.

O 13

Because the patient is lying in bed for long periods of time during dialysis, skin breakdown over the pressure points can occur rapidly. Additional factors contributing to this problem are the uremic skin symptoms and the lethargy renal patients frequently experience.

I 3, 14

Problems with neurologic functioning are not common during peritoneal dialysis, but the ordinary observations of consciousness and thought processes should be maintained. ECG monitoring is not routine unless the patient has cardiac problems.

In addition to making these observations during dialysis, a number of nursing interventions are important to the success of the procedure and the patient's comfort.

## Nursing Interventions During Peritoneal Dialysis

*Problem 4*

Choose the nursing interventions that will increase the patient's comfort during the procedure. Squares numbered: ____________

*Problem 5*

Now list the nursing actions that will directly prevent the secondary complications of pneumonia, skin breakdown, venous stasis, infection, and a catabolic state. Squares numbered: ____________

*Problem 6*

Dialysate removed during the drainage time should equal or exceed the volume infused. If less is gotten back, what nursing actions should be taken? Squares numbered: ____________

*Problem 7*

Which of the interventions are related to organizing nursing care to accomplish the dialysis procedure. Squares numbered: ____________

| Response Indicator | | | | |
|---|---|---|---|---|
| Constant awareness of the exact status of the exchange 1 | Consistent recording of fluid balance 2 | Accurate timing of phases of dialysis 3 | Warming of dialysate to 37°C 4 | Having patient cough and hyperventilate frequently 5 |
| Changing of position from side to side frequently 6 | Massage of body prominances with lotion 7 | Raising head of bed 8 | Administering analgesics and Xylocaine as ordered 9 | Encouraging intake of protein in diet 10 |
| Strict aseptic technique in handling infusion set and catheter site 11 | Leg exercises and elastic hose 12 | Gentle massage of abdomen 13 | Providing diversionary activities; visitors, TV, reading 14 | Explaining things about the procedure that patient needs or wants to know 15 |

| Response Indicator | | | | |
|---|---|---|---|---|
| Constant awareness of the exact status of the exchange 1 | Consistent recording of fluid balance 2 | Accurate timing of phases of dialysis 3 | Warming of dialysate to 37°C 4 | Having patient cough and hyperventilate frequently 5 |
| Changing of position from side to side frequently 6 | Massage of body prominances with lotion 7 | Raising head of bed 8 | Administering analgesics and Xylocaine as ordered 9 | Encouraging intake of protein in diet 10 |
| Strict aseptic technique in handling infusion set and catheter site 11 | Leg exercises and elastic hose 12 | Gentle massage of abdomen 13 | Providing diversionary activities; visitors, TV, reading 14 | Explaining things about the procedure that patient needs or wants to know 15 |

## Comments

*Problem 4* — Patient's Comfort

Suggested responses: 4, 6, 7, 8, 9, 14, 15

These are correct because: warming the dialysate prevents pain and chilling on instillation; change of position and back-rubs help during periods of relative immobility; analgesics should be used as needed; and diversionary activities and appropriate patient teaching provide psychologic comfort. The leg exercises and elastic hose (12) may be a comfort measure to some patients. The abdominal massage (13) is to promote drainage and may be uncomfortable.

*Problem 5* — Secondary Complications

Suggested responses: 5, 6, 7, 8, 10, 11, 12

Coughing, hyperventilation and position changes help to aerate all portions of the lungs and prevent pneumonia; change in position and massage prevent skin breakdown; leg exercises and elastic hose prevent venous stasis and clotting; aseptic technique prevents infection; and encouragement of dietary intake of protein would replace protein losses during dialysis.

*Problem 6* — Poor Catheter Drainage

Suggested responses: 6, 8, 13

These interventions would help to free the catheter tip so it could drain and adds hydrostatic pressure to encourage drainage. Another possibility here would be that the catheter is plugged with a clot or fibrin. Heparin irrigation or use of a stylet to clear the catheter lumen may then be needed.

*Problem 7* — Organization of Nursing Care

Suggested responses: 1, 2, 3, 4

These are all important in the nursing management of the dialysis procedure and require organization of time and tasks.

## Assisting the patient to cope with treatment

Suzanne and her husband had many questions about peritoneal dialysis, the planned switch to chronic hemodialysis, and the possibility of kidney transplantation. Her needs for information and counseling were met by the interdisciplinary team responsible for her care. This group included Ellen—her primary nurse, her physicians, the social worker, and her minister. Ellen completed a patient education assessment (see Appendix C and D) and the group developed a teaching plan with Ellen.

To pass the time faster, Suzanne began working at her hobby of sketching. She had taken some art courses and enjoyed making original designs for notepaper. One day she showed Ellen this sketch, saying, "This is my self portrait."

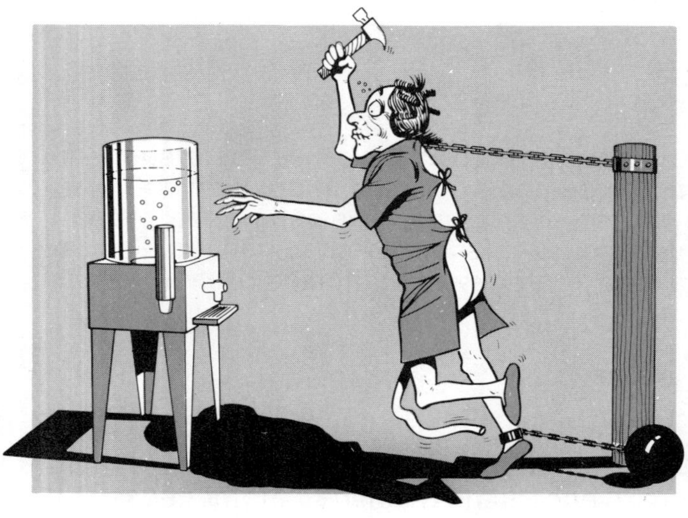

Figure 49

### Frame 19

What do you think Suzanne was trying to express about herself in this drawing?

Your choice (Probably difficulty with fluid restriction, problems with body image changes, maybe a feeling of being trapped)

## Frame 20

Ellen said, "You've drawn yourself in a pretty miserable position."

"Yes," Suzanne replied, "Just knowing that you aren't supposed to drink makes you all the more thirsty . . . it is miserable . . . just look at me, yellow, dried up, with this big tube hanging out in front. How will my clothes fit? Don will be ashamed of me. It seems that this time in the hospital is endless. The bills will ruin us, and the future is so uncertain."

Which of these is the best interpretation of Suzanne's remarks?

a. She is depressed and suicidal
b. They are an example of humor as a denial mechanism
c. They are an appropriate response to her situation

c

## Frame 21

What approach(es) should Ellen take?

a. Encourage Suzanne to identify and talk with the team members who can help (for example, social worker for financial worries)
b. Explain that life has a higher priority than physical appearance
c. Reassure her that her husband will not be ashamed of her
d. Accept her concerns as important issues
e. Arrange for Suzanne to talk with patients who are successfully managing chronic dialysis
f. Suggest a patient and family team conference

a, d, e, maybe f

After three weeks of hospitalization, Suzanne went home. She returned to the hospital three times a week for a 10-hour peritoneal dialysis with an automatic machine until her hemodialysis fistula was ready for use.

## Frame 22

Here is a list of advantages and disadvantages of peritoneal dialysis:

*Advantages*

1. Simple equipment, can be done in any hospital
2. Can be initiated quickly
3. No need for systemic anticoagulants with hazards of hemorrhage
4. Slower dialysis with less risk of hypotension, embolism, and hepatitis

*Disadvantages*

1. Time-consuming
2. Protein loss
3. Discomfort for patient
4. Risk of peritonitis, pneumonia

Which of the disadvantages can be minimized by excellent nursing care?

3, 4

## Frame 23

Summary:

The nursing care involved in preparing the patient for peritoneal dialysis includes teaching the patient what to expect, gathering a data baseline for assessing progress of the procedure (weight, blood pressure, pulse, and temperature), making sure that the patient voids, and setting up the equipment.

During the procedure the nurse observes fluid balance by following the input and output record, weight, blood pressure, and pulse. Laboratory tests provide for observing solute balances. The nurse also observes for symptoms of complications due to fluid and electrolyte imbalances.

Nursing interventions include providing comfort measures and helping recover fluid during the drain phase. Other nursing actions help prevent complications such as pneumonia, peritonitis, skin breakdown, and venous stasis.

The successful outcome of peritoneal dialysis is directly affected by knowledgeable, organized nursing care.

See Appendix B for nursing care plan information.

# CHAPTER 14
## ACUTE RENAL FAILURE

A variety of events and agents can lead to a sudden drop in urinary flow and to the numerous clinical symptoms resulting from renal failure. In Chapter 2 the prerenal causes such as shock, decreased cardiac output, and altered renal circulation were discussed. Acute renal failure develops rapidly (in hours to days) and there is a chance of reversing the damage with proper treatment. If acute failure is reversed, normal urine output will be reestablished in several weeks or months. Roger Jamison's complicated course after a ruptured abdominal aortic aneurysm is an example of acute renal failure.

After completing this chapter, you will be able to

1. Recognize the relationship between the hemodynamic events in shock and acute renal failure
2. Develop assessment priorities for a specific clinical situation
3. Relate specific modalities of treatment to the goals of care
4. Choose nursing interventions that would help a patient cope with crisis
5. Describe the clinical picture of the oliguric and diuretic phases of acute tubular necrosis.

# CASE PRESENTATION

## PART I
## THE PRECIPITATING EVENT

It was a Saturday forenoon in May. Sixty-year-old Roger Jamison was relaxing at home after a busy week as a bank treasurer. He was building on his wood-working project. As he lifted a board he developed very sharp pains in his lower abdomen and both groins. His wife helped him get into bed to rest. He was frightened but kept thinking, "I've just pulled a muscle." He decided he must lose some weight and get back into shape. As he rested in bed, he said, "I feel like I am going to pass out." At last his wife called an ambulance to rush him to see his doctor. Even by ambulance, it took over an hour to get to the hospital.

Mr. Jamison arrived at the emergency room about 4 hours after the onset of his pain. His blood pressure was 60–100/?, pulse 100 and regular. He complained of having persistent right lower quadrant pain and diarrhea. He was slightly dyspneic. The abdomen was large, distended, and rigid, and bowel sounds were absent.

Within an hour, Mr. Jamison had received 1,250 ml of Plasmanate and 1,500 ml of lactated Ringer's solution. Since his blood pressure did not stabilize in response to this volume expansion, he also was receiving a metaraminol bitartrate (Aramine) drip. The ECG monitor showed a normal sinus rhythm. A urinary catheter was inserted and urinary output was scant—only a few ml's in the tubing. A surgeon had also examined him and he was prepared for an emergency exploratory laparotomy.

During the laparotomy, a ruptured abdominal aortic aneurysm was repaired with a Dacron graft. The estimated blood loss was 12,000 ml. Whole blood replacement was 11,000 ml, plus 600 ml fresh frozen plasma and 1,250 ml Plasmanate.

Mr. Jamison's blood pressure dropped as low as 40–60/? and he was anuric for several hours. Methylprednisolone sodium succinate (Solu-Medrol), furosemide (Lasix), and mannitol were given to improve his urinary output. Levarterenol bitartrate (Levophed), isoproterenol (Isuprel), sodium bicarbonate, and calcium chloride were also used to correct problems due to the prolonged period of shock. During the last 2 hours of surgery his kidneys began making urine at about 600 ml/hour. His blood pressure at the time of leaving the operating room was 140/90, pulse 112. Because the surgical area continued to bleed, his abdomen was packed with Gelfoam and two drains connected to disposable suction devices were inserted prior to closure. Over 10 hours after the onset of pain, Roger Jamison was admitted to the surgical intensive care unit.

# DISCUSSION

## Frame 1

Mr. Jamison's shock state was caused by which of the following?

a. Peritonitis
b. Hypovolemia
c. Cardiac pump failure
d. Increased peripheral vascular resistance

b

## Frame 2

Plasmanate is a solution that contains plasma proteins. Lactated Ringer's is an isotonic solution containing electrolytes. Choose the correct statements about the treatment of hypovolemia:

a. These solutions were used to expand the blood volume on a temporary basis.
b. During surgery whole blood and plasma were used to replace lost blood.
c. Mr. Jamison received too much fluid.
d. The blood pressure is an indication of the adequacy of circulating blood volume.

a, b, d

## Frame 3

Mr. Jamison's systolic blood pressure dropped below the range in which kidney autoregulation of perfusion pressure is effective. Much less blood flowed through the glomerular capillaries. This would cause:

1. Glomerular filtration rate to (increase/decrease).

1. decrease because of decreased blood flow through the glomerulus.

2. Amount of filtrate in the proximal tubule (increases/decreases).

2. decreases

The lower volume of filtrate flows more slowly through the tubule, as it is under lower pressure. There is more time for sodium and water reabsorption. This would cause:

3. Urine volume (increases/decreases).

3. decreases

4. Specific gravity would be (higher/lower).

4. higher (Solutes are present with less water.)

## Frame 4

Because prolonged oliguria can cause renal tissue damage, drugs are frequently given to increase output.

*Furosemide* (Lasix) is frequently used to increase the amount of water excreted.

*Mannitol* is a form of mannose sugar. It is filtered by the glomerulus but not reabsorbed by the tubule. Its presence in the filtrate exerts an osmotic effect, which keeps water in the tubule and thereby increases output.

If the patient's urinary output increases with the use of these drugs, the renal failure is thought to be reversible.

Mark the following statements true or false:

1. ______ Prolonged oliguria has no long-term effects on renal tissue.

1. False

2. ______ Mr. Jamison's oliguria is related to his low glomerular filtration rate during shock.

2. True

3. ______ Furosemide and mannitol are given to concentrate the urine.

3. False (These dilute the urine, as more water is excreted.)

4. ______ Mr. Jamison's renal response to furosemide and mannitol indicates that his renal failure is reversible.

4. True

## Frame 5

Several of the drugs used to treat Mr. Jamison's shock state may further decrease kidney perfusion. Metaraminol bitartrate (Aramine) and Levarterenol bitartrate (Levophed) are peripheral vasoconstrictors.

Decreasing the size of blood vessels compensates for low blood volume and increases systemic blood pressure. Because these drugs also constrict the renal artery, the blood flow to the kidney is reduced even more. These drugs are usually given only as an emergency measure in hypovolemic shock, until the blood volume is replaced.

Mark these statements true or false:

1. ______ Systemic blood pressure is always an indication of adequate renal perfusion.
2. ______ Vasoconstrictors can decrease the glomerular filtration rate.
3. ______ Mr. Jamison's urinary output is an accurate indication of his renal perfusion.

1. False
2. True
3. True (If perfusion pressure is not adequate for filtration, output decreases.)

# CASE PRESENTATION
# PART II
# THE OLIGURIC PHASE

During the period immediately following shock, renal perfusion may still be decreased, and it may take time for normal urinary output to be established. However, if damage to the tubular cells has occurred, oliguria will persist.

When Mr. Jamison was admitted to ICU, Jill Renning was assigned as his nurse.

Here is Jill's admission note:

1. Vital Signs:
   BP 110/80, P-104, R – 12, T 96.4 °F
   Weight—190 pounds
2. Cardiac:
   Heart tones clear, no murmur or rub. ECG monitor shows regular sinus rhythm.
3. Respiratory:
   Color pale, no dyspnea, normal chest excursions, lung sounds clear and heard in each lobe, cyanosis of extremities.
4. Neural:
   Patient responds to name, follows commands to move all extremities, pupils equal and react to light, hand grasps equal and strong.
5. Renal:
   Foley catheter in place, 700 ml clear yellow urine in bag.
6. Gastrointestinal:
   N.G. tube to low intermittent suction, returns—scant dark red mucus, abdomen rounded, soft, and silent.
7. Skin:
   Skin cool and dry.
8. Extremities:
   Upper—circulation ok. Left arterial line—D5W—3 ml/hr, to keep line open
   Right arm—D5W in ½ N.S.—100 ml/hr.

   Lower—color of feet and legs dusky to cyanotic, bilaterally palpable pedal and popliteal pulses.
9. Wound:
   Two wound drains—180 ml of bright red drainage. Incisional dressings present, dry.

# DISCUSSION

The next response indicator provides a list of many observations important in Roger's care. We want you to set some priorities among these by deciding which ones should be constantly in Jill's awareness; and which need to be documented at frequent intervals, and at longer intervals.

*Problem 1*

Use the Response Indicator to construct a list of parameters Jill should monitor and record continuously. Squares numbered: ______________

*Problem 2*

Now identify the observations to be made and recorded every 1–2 hours. Squares numbered: ______________

*Problem 3*

If Roger's condition remains stable, which observations could be made and documented once or twice each shift? Squares numbered: ______________

| Response Indicator | | | | |
|---|---|---|---|---|
| Pulse: Apical<br>Radial<br>Popliteal<br>Pedal<br>1 | Cardiac rhythm<br>2 | Temperature<br>3 | Breath sounds<br>4 | Heart sounds<br>5 |
| Arterial blood pressure<br>6 | Respirations–rate and quality; skin color<br>7 | Bleeding from wound drains and incision<br>8 | Urinary output<br>9 | Neuro checks<br>10 |
| Abdominal inspection and palpation<br>11 | Nasogastric tube drainage<br>12 | Hgb.<br>Hct.<br>Platelets<br>Bleeding time<br>13 | BUN creatinine<br>14 | Serum electrolytes<br>15 |
| Blood gases<br>16 | Color, skin temperature and sensation of legs<br>17 | | | |

| Response Indicator | | | | |
|---|---|---|---|---|
| Pulse: Apical Radial Popliteal Pedal 1 | Cardiac rhythm 2 | Temperature 3 | Breath sounds 4 | Heart sounds 5 |
| Arterial blood pressure 6 | Respirations-rate and quality; skin color 7 | Bleeding from wound drains and incision 8 | Urinary output 9 | Neuro checks 10 |
| Abdominal inspection and palpation 11 | Nasogastric tube drainage 12 | Hgb. Hct. Platelets Bleeding time 13 | BUN creatinine 14 | Serum electrolytes 15 |
| Blood gases 16 | Color, skin temperature and sensation of legs 17 | | | |

## Comments

*Problem 1* — Continuous Monitoring

Suggested responses: 1, 2, 6, 7, and 8

O 1, 2, 6, 7

These observations are the highest priority as they indicate the adequacy of tissue perfusion and hemodynamic stability. Significant changes in any of these parameters would be the first signs of deepening shock, cardiac insufficiency, disruption and/or clotting of the graft and distal vascular system. These developments would require immediate medical intervention.

O 8

Since Mr. Jamison had extensive intraabdominal bleeding, Jill would expect some wound drainage. However, very close observation is required since the bleeding may not be stopped and Roger is barely out of hypovolemic shock.

*Problem 2* — Observations Made Hourly

Suggested responses: 9, 10, 11, and 17

I 1, 2, 6, 7, 8

These observations belong under continuous monitoring.

O 9, 10, 11, 17

Each of these parameters is important enough to be observed at least every hour. Jill would want to record hourly urine output, since 20–30 ml must be produced each hour to adequately clear wastes from the blood.

Mr. Jamison will probably have periods of sleep due to lingering effects of anesthesia. During wakeful periods, neuro checks should be done.

| Response Indicator | | | | |
|---|---|---|---|---|
| Pulse: Apical Radial Popli-teal Pedal 1 | Cardiac rhythm 2 | Temperature 3 | Breath sounds 4 | Heart sounds 5 |
| Arterial blood pressure 6 | Respirations-rate and quality; skin color 7 | Bleeding from wound drains and incision 8 | Urinary output 9 | Neuro checks 10 |
| Abdominal inspection and palpation 11 | Nasogastric tube drainage 12 | Hgb. Hct. Platelets Bleeding time 3 | BUN creatinine 14 | Serum electrolytes 15 |
| Blood gases 16 | Color, skin temperature and sensation of legs 17 | | | |

Intraabdominal bleeding will cause distention and rigidity of the abdomen.

Observing color, temperature, and sensation of the legs gives an indication of the integrity of the graft and patency of circulation.

*Problem 3* — Observations Made Every 4–8 Hours

Suggested Responses: 3, 4, 5, 12, 13, 14, 15, 16

I 1, 2, 6, 7, 8, 9, 10, 11, 17

All of these observations should be made more often.

O 3, 4, 5

If the patient's pulse, cardiac rhythm, blood pressure, and respirations are monitored continuously, Jill can add auscultation of the chest and temperature to her assessment at longer intervals. Sometimes it is impossible to see all and do all, so priorities need to be identified to keep the situation manageable.

O 13, 14, 15, 16

These lab tests may be ordered more or less often, depending on the patient's condition. Jill would need to be knowledgeable about the latest lab values and their relationship to her assessment.

# CASE PRESENTATION

From 11 PM to 3 AM, Mr. Jamison's care revolved around active bleeding from the abdominal drains which caused hypotension. He required whole blood transfusions and IV protamine to try to slow the blood loss of 175 ml/hour. His urine output had decreased after the large diuresis to about 50 ml/hour. There was no increased urinary response to 20 mg IV furosemide (Lasix). Mr. Jamison continued to be alert; he was anxious and restless.

In the morning the surgeon decided to have a renal consult. After Mr. Jamison was seen by the nephrologist, a renogram was done to rule out the possibility of the anuria being caused by an obstruction. There was decreased renal perfusion but no obstruction. The nephrologist ordered increasing dosages of furosemide (Lasix 80mg–160mg–240mg–1 g) and urine output was maintained at about 50–100 ml/hour. Digoxin was begun to improve cardiac output.

The chief goals of the medical treatment plan for Mr. Jamison were

1. Replace blood volume
2. Repair the disrupted vascular system
3. Balance body water and electrolytes
4. Maintain urinary output.

Mr. Jamison's intraabdominal bleeding was gradually ceasing but because of this problem, the physicians decided to avoid hemodialysis as long as possible. Blood losses were replaced ml for ml by whole blood. Platelets were given to keep an adequate level. Vitamin K, 5 mg IM was given because it is important in the formation of blood clotting factors. Magaldrate (Riopan) 15 ml/NG was given every 2 hours with a 15-minute clamp time to prevent stress ulcers. Nasogastric returns were not replaced because of a need to keep fluid intake down. Blood studies that were followed were: Hgb., Hct., platelets, and bleeding time. Stools were tested for presence of blood.

Mr. Jamison was then transferred to the renal intensive care unit, as the acute renal failure was considered his most important problem. The treatment plan was geared toward trying to increase the renal output, maintain fluid and electrolyte balance, support protein anabolism and wound healing, and maintain circulatory adequacy.

# DISCUSSION

Now look at the specific methods used to evaluate and treat Mr. Jamison's problems. The Response Indicator lists these orders, and you will relate them to the treatment goals.

*Problem 1*

Which orders are related to *maintaining* and *assessing* fluid balance? Squares numbered: ______________

*Problem 2*

Which orders are directed toward *maintaining* and *assessing* electrolyte balance? Squares numbered: ______________

*Problem 3*

How is the urinary output being maintained? Squares numbered: ______________

*Problem 4*

Because of the bleeding, tissue damage and lack of oral intake, protein homeostasis was identified as a problem. How is this being dealt with? Squares numbered: ______________

| Response Indicator | | |
|---|---|---|
| Furosemide (Lasix) IM 80–160 mg. 1 | Daily weight 2 | IV's at 100 ml/hour Decrease to 50 ml/hour if pulmonary wedge pressure is below 15 3 |
| BP qh 4 | Record: Intake Output (urine, blood, NG secretion) 5 | Total parenteral nutrition with a solution high in dextrose, low in potassium and with a small amount of essential amino acids 6 |
| Pulmonary wedge pressure monitoring 7 | Kayexalate retention enemas for serum K over 6 mEq/L 8 | Serum electrolytes 9 |
| EKG monitoring 10 | | |

| Response Indicator | | |
|---|---|---|
| Furosemide (Lasix) IM 80-160 mg. 1 | Daily weight 2 | IV's at 100 ml/hour Decrease to 50 ml/hour if pulmonary wedge pressure is below 15 3 |
| BP qh 4 | Record: Intake Output (urine, blood, NG secretion) 5 | Total parenteral nutrition with a solution high in dextrose, low in potassium and with a small amount of essential amino acids 6 |
| Pulmonary wedge pressure monitoring 7 | Kayexalate retention enemas for serum K over 6 mEq/L 8 | Serum electrolytes 9 |
| EKG monitoring 10 | | |

## Comments

*Problem 1* — Fluid Balance

Suggested responses: 1, 2, 3, 4, 5, 6 and 7

O 2, 4, 5, 7

These are all assessment parameters important in judging fluid balance. High intake and low output, along with increased weight, blood pressure, and pulmonary wedge pressure, indicate impending fluid overload.

O 1, 3, 6

IVs and TPN are the chief sources of fluid intake. These contain varying combinations of solutes, and the rate of administration is regulated to meet the fluid and electrolyte requirements of the body.

*Problem 2* — Electrolyte Balance

Suggested responses: 3, 6, 8, 9 and 10

O 8

Kayexalate is a powdered cation resin. As it is retained in the colon after the enema, it exchanges its sodium ions for potassium ions, thereby lowering serum potassium levels. (Kayexalate may also be taken orally if the patient can tolerate it.)

O 9, 10

The electrolyte levels can be followed by blood tests. It is particularly important to watch Mr. Jamison's potassium and sodium levels. In acute renal failure, the kidney is not able to excrete excess potassium. High blood levels are dangerous as cardiac arrhythmias can result. Sodium levels must also be regulated, especially when potent diuretics such as furosemide (Lasix) are used.

The ECG tracing can give indications of the cardiotoxic effects of high potassium levels. (See Chapter 5, Frames 24–27 for specific information.)

O 3, 6

The IVs and TPN are the chief mode of intake of electrolytes.

| Response Indicator | | |
|---|---|---|
| Furosemide (Lasix) IM 80–160 mg. 1 | Daily weight 2 | IV's at [illegible]00 ml/hour Decrease to 50 ml/hour if pulmonary wedge pressure is below [illegible]5 3 |
| BP qh 4 | Record: Intake Output (urine, blood, NG secretion) 5 | Total parenteral nutrition with a solution high in dextrose, low in potassium and with a small amount of essential amino acids 6 |
| Pulmonary wedge pressure monitoring 7 | Kayexalate retention enemas for serum K over 6 mEq/L 8 | Serum electrolytes 9 |
| EKG monitoring 10 | | |

*Problem 3* — Urinary Output

Suggested responses: 1 and 3

O 1, 3

Furosemide (Lasix) is a potent diuretic, given to decrease the reabsorption of sodium and water by the tubule, and thereby, to increase output. IV fluids stimulate output by maintaining adequate blood volume and renal perfusion pressure.

*Problem 4* — Protein Homeostasis

Suggested response: 6

O 6

Total parenteral nutrition provides a nutrient solution with high glucose content. The glucose is metabolized to meet the energy requirements of the body, thus sparing protein. The protein can then be used to build up tissues and heal wounds. The solution also contains electrolytes and trace elements, as well as protein, for adequate total nutrition.

# CASE PRESENTATION PART III REACTION TO CRISIS

Ellen noticed that Mr. Jamison was restless and anxious since his transfer to the renal unit. He was irritated with procedures and tests; and spoke only to voice complaints of pain, discomfort, and dissatisfaction with the care he was receiving.

The group of physicians responsible for Mr. Jamison's care had just made rounds and spent considerable time examining him, discussing the diagnostic data, and deciding the next step in their treatment plan. Mr. Jamison listened to this with close attention, and when the group left he exploded in anger, saying to Ellen

> *"I'm sick and tired of the incompetence of you people. Here I am, sick—maybe even dying—and all you do is take blood tests, look at that urine bag, and talk. I want something done! They say I have kidney failure. That doesn't make sense. I have never had a bit of trouble with my kidneys in my whole life. My wife is no help, she just comes in here and says, 'Don't fuss—be glad you're alive.' Well, I probably won't be alive much longer if you people don't get on the ball and do something to cure me."*

Ellen said, "You feel that you are seriously ill and not enough is being done to help you, is that right?" Mr. Jamison nodded, trying to hold back tears. Then he said

> *"Why did this have to happen to me? I am at the age now when I can think about retiring and enjoying the life I've planned for. There are so many things I want to do. I've always taken good care of my health. I can't believe this is really happening to me."*

# DISCUSSION

## Frame 6

Which of the following approaches should Ellen use to help Mr. Jamison deal with his feelings?

a. Explain that his care has been excellent and that he is lucky to have come through this crisis as well as he has
b. Give him some patient education information to read about renal failure, and offer to discuss it with him
c. Acknowledge and accept his feelings of anger
d. Win him over by cheerfulness and humor.
e. Show him that you realize what a difficult situation he is in
f. Arrange for other nurses to care for him, since Ellen makes him angry and he thinks she is incompetent
g. Carefully explain the purpose of procedures and tests
h. Encourage verbal expression of anger
i. Anticipate his needs

c, e, g, h, and i are the best responses. For further discussion:
a, d—see Frame 7
b, g—see Frame 8
c, e, h, i—see Frame 9
f—see Frame 10

## Frame 7 (a, d)

These two approaches would probably not be helpful to Mr. Jamison. Expressing the opinion that he is lucky and that his care is excellent directly contradicts what he was saying and may make him more angry. He might interpret cheerfulness and humor as evidence of lack of caring or recognition of the gravity of his situation.

## Frame 8 (b, g)

There is a difference between approaches b and g. It is important that Mr. Jamison is given a careful explanation of the purpose of procedures and tests (g), so that he can give informed consent and cooperation. However, he probably is not ready for reading patient education materials. He is expressing shock and disbelief about the whole thing—which is a common initial reaction to crisis. When a person feels this way, he or she is usually not open to learning intellectual facts. Patients like Mr. Jamison often signal their readiness for explanation by verbal (and nonverbal) requests for more information about specific aspects of care.

### Frame 9 (c, e, h, i)

Approaches c, e, and h would acknowledge the real seriousness of the situation and Mr. Jamison's right to feel angry about it. He would get the message that he is respected and that Ellen is trying to understand his viewpoint. By anticipating his needs, she will demonstrate her caring and competence.

### Frame 10 (f)

This approach is avoidance behavior by the nurse and might further increase Mr. Jamison's hostility and sense of isolation. Occasionally, a nurse may find his or her personality clashing with a patient's and withdrawal is appropriate. But in this situation, Mr. Jamison seems to be lashing out at everyone because he is really afraid. Some of the approaches outlined above would be much more helpful.

# CASE PRESENTATION PART IV ACUTE TUBULAR NECROSIS

On the 3rd postop day, Mr. Jamison's 12-hour creatinine clearance was 5 ml/min and serum creatinine was 7.5 mg/100 ml. (Normals: Ccr = 85–125, Scr = 0–1) The next day his serum creatinine rose to 8.9 mg/100 ml, and BUN was 90 mg/100 ml. It was harder to control the serum potassium with Kayexalate. His urine output was no longer responsive to large doses of furosemide (Lasix) and hourly outputs averaged 20 ml. In addition his temperature had been rising since surgery, and was now 103°F. The source of sepsis was unknown at this time. The one positive sign was that his bleeding had slowed considerably and was now less than 10 ml/hour.

The physicians added antibiotics to the IVs to treat the infectious process. They used the creatinine clearance data to calculate dosages of gentamicin 200 mg daily and ampicillin 1 g every 4 hours. The reason for extra care in this matter is that some antibiotics, such as gentamicin, can have nephrotoxic side effects.

Because of the decrease in urine output, the rising BUN, the uncontrolled serum potassium and some signs of fluid overload, the physicians decided to begin hemodialysis.

# PART V
# THE DIURETIC AND RECOVERY PHASE

After 2 weeks on hemodialysis, Mr. Jamison's urine output began to increase gradually with an average of 50 ml/day. On some days it was less than this, but the amount would increase the next day. The wound bleeding had stopped, hemodynamic stability returned, and total parenteral nutrition (hyperalimentation) was discontinued as soon as he could eat an adequate diet.

The doctors wanted to decrease the amount of dialyzing time, but Mr. Jamison's BUN and potassium were still increasing rapidly between dialysis treatments. In another week this seemed to stabilize, and Mr. Jamison was dialyzed only when necessary. The first interval was 4 days, but then he needed dialysis to decrease electrolytes and metabolic wastes which had built up. By this time, his urine output was about 1,000 ml/day with specific gravities between 1.005 and 1.010. His oral intake of fluid had to be at least 500 ml more than the amount of urine output. Patients who are not on dialysis may have intense diuresis during this stage of renal failure, because the healing tubule cells are not able to reabsorb all the water and sodium. Attention is then given to prevention of dehydration and sodium depletion.

Seven weeks after rupture of his abdominal aneurysm Mr. Jamison was ready to go home. He had needed two more hemodialysis treatments. Then the cannula was tied off and removed. His urine output averaged about 1,200 ml/day, his BUN was 28 mg/100 ml, and creatinine, 1.9 mg/100 ml. A creatinine clearance was 50 ml/min. Mr. Jamison was given an appointment to return to the renal clinic in 2 weeks. He was to bring with him a 24-hour urine collection for clearance tests.

For the next six months, Mr. Jamison returned to the clinic monthly. His creatinine clearance rose to about 75 ml/min but there was no problem with how his kidneys handled the fluids and solutes. He described his health as "pretty good," and was able to enjoy the retirement he had planned.

You will learn more about Mr. Jamison's dialysis treatments in the following chapter.

Summary:

Acute renal failure is the result of necrosis of the epithelial cells of the renal tubule which is brought on by renal ischemia or nephrotoxic chemicals.

It progresses in three stages:

1. Oliguric phase—oliguria leading to anuria and rapidly progressing azotemia
2. Diuretic phase—regeneration of tubule cells accompanied by diuresis due to lack of concentrating ability in the new cells. Azotemia continues.
3. Recovery phase—reestablishment of tubular function and adequate clearances, which may require months.

Shock is a frequent cause of acute renal failure in critical care units.

Shock is inadequacy of circulating blood volume, with decreased tissue perfusion.

Decreased perfusion in glomeruli results in decreased volume of filtrate and necrosis of renal tubules.

Treatment goals are to increase effective circulating volume and maintain urinary output of 20–30 ml/hour, reflecting adequate renal perfusion.

Treatment methods include volume replacement and/or expansion, diuretics, vasopressors (which may decrease renal perfusion), and vasodilators.

Nursing Care

See sample nursing care plan in Appendix B, Problems I, II, III, IV, V, VI, VII, VIII, XI, XVI, and XVII.

# CHAPTER 15

## HEMODIALYSIS

### Introduction

Hemodialysis is the use of a specially designed machine to perform the work of the kidneys. Years of experience with this procedure have made it a safe and frequently prescribed treatment. *You would need a special course to learn how to run a dialysis machine and care for the patient during treatment.* But, after completing this chapter, you will be able to

1. List the indications for hemodialysis
2. Differentiate between the two basic types of access for hemodialysis
3. List advantages and disadvantages of each type of access
4. Define an "arterialized vein"
5. Describe the nursing care related to access sites
6. Identify potential complications during and after dialysis
7. Identify the four components of any hemodialyzer
8. Label examples of the three basic types of currently used hemodialyzers
9. Design a plan for nursing care of the patient after dialysis
10. List four methods used to prevent hepatitis.

### Chapter outline

- Uses of hemodialysis
- Access to circulation
  - External
    - Temporary
    - Permanent
  - Internal
- Procedure
  - Connection
  - Dialysis process
  - Equipment
  - Physical complications
- Nursing care of patients following dialysis

# PART I
# USES OF HEMODIALYSIS

In chapter 14 you looked at the clinical course of Roger Jamison. He had hypovolemic shock which caused acute renal failure, and he was treated with hemodialysis. This chapter will refer to his dialysis experiences.

## Frame 1

Hemodialysis is one of the alternatives considered when dialysis is indicated.

Hemodialysis is particularly needed if

1. The patient has had extensive abdominal surgery or infection, which would contraindicate peritoneal dialysis
2. A rapid change of fluid and/or chemical level is desired
3. An efficient, less time-consuming procedure is desired.

Of the three reasons for hemodialysis, choose the ones you feel apply to Mr. Jamison's case:

See Frame 2 for answer.

## Frame 2

1, 2, and possibly 3.

1. Mr. Jamison had had extensive abdominal surgery, which contraindicates peritoneal dialysis.
2. Correcting the increasing hypervolemia and controlling hyperkalemia were the major reasons to initiate dialysis.
3. Number 3 probably was also a consideration, although from the data given, you are not able to know for sure.

# PART II ACCESS TO CIRCULATION

## External Type

Today's use of hemodialysis was made possible by the development of ways to repeatedly gain access to the patient's circulatory system. A hemodialysis access is either completely *internal* (subcutaneous) or has an *external* device.

First look at an external device, the Shaldon femoral catheter which is a *temporary* method of access, to be used once or twice until a permanent access can be created.

Shaldon catheters can be used in two ways:

1. Figure 50 shows two catheters placed in the femoral vein. Blood is removed via the "arterial" catheter, run through a dialysis machine for purification, and returned by means of another femoral catheter.

VASCULAR ACCESS VIA SHALDON CATHETERS

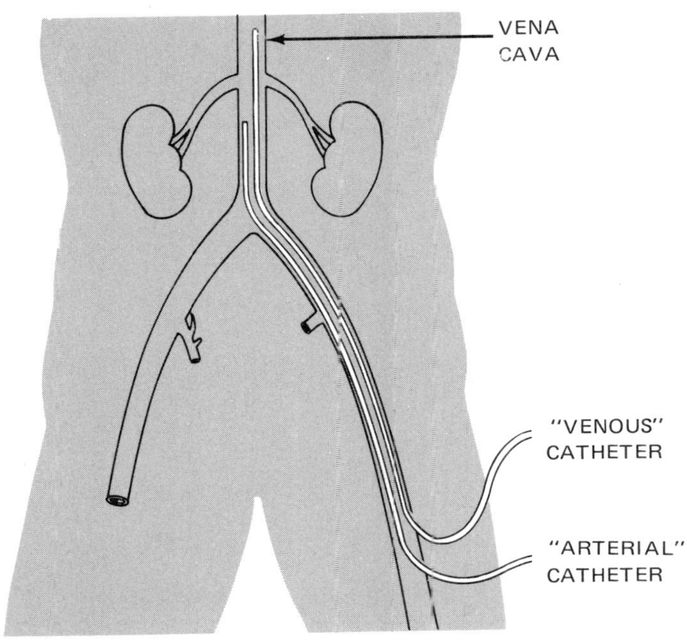


Figure 50

2. In Mr. Jamison's case, one catheter is placed in the femoral vein and the blood is returned via an indwelling intravenous catheter in an arm vein. When the Shaldon catheter is left in place and when it is removed, care must be taken to prevent hemorrhage.

## Frame 3

Considering the placement of the Shaldon catheter, which of these activities could kink or dislodge it?

b, c

a. Bed rest
b. Bathroom privileges
c. Riding in a wheelchair
d. Repositioning without bending the groin (log rolling)

*Panel 1*

*The next morning, a* permanent *external access was placed in Mr. Jamison's left radial artery and cephalic vein. This was used for the rest of his dialysis treatments.*

*This figure shows one kind of external arteriovenous shunt (a cannula) which is often used. Notice that Teflon tips are sewn into a vein and an artery. The tips are attached to Silastic tubing which is brought to the surface of the skin to make an external connection between the blood vessels. The plastic connector in the tubing is used to open the shunt for connection to the dialysis machine tubing.*

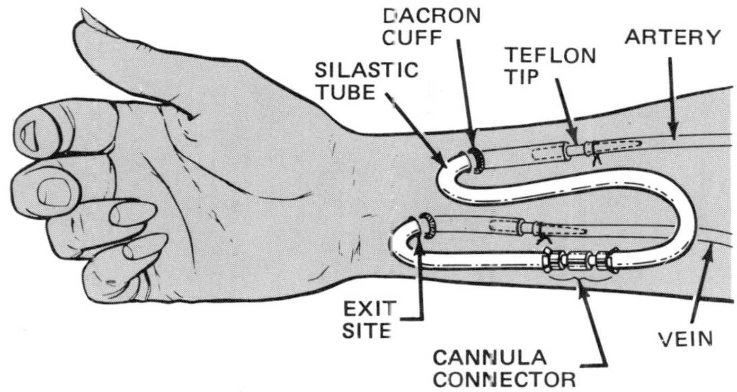


Figure 51

*A shunt is placed in a procedure called a* cannulation. *It is similar to a cut-down procedure. Shunts can be placed in either the arm or the leg.*

*After a local anesthetic, one or two incisions are made to locate an artery and a nearby vein of appropriate size. The blood vessels are ligated and the shunt tips inserted and secured into place with sutures.*

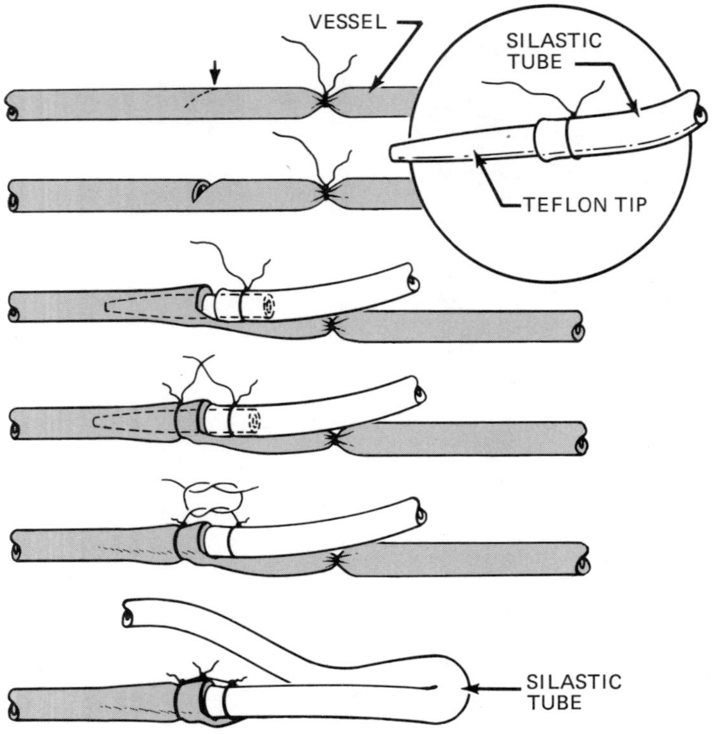


Figure 52

*The Silastic tubes are then brought to the outside through punctured holes in the skin* (the exit sites). *The tubing is joined by a special connector and when a good blood flow has been established, the incisions are closed.*

Advantages

*Can be readily placed*

*May be used immediately for dialysis*

*No venipunctures for each dialysis*

Disadvantages

*One site may only last several months*

*More incidence of infection—the skin around the exit sites does not adhere to the tubing*

*More incidence of clotting*

*Danger of tubing separation resulting in hemorrhage*

*Restricted movement of extremity*

*Daily dressing changes with skin care*

## Frame 4

Special plastics (Silastic and Teflon) are used to make external shunts. The surfaces are smooth and do not absorb moisture, therefore, they help prevent clotting. A disadvantage is that the plastic will not reseal if punctured. Decide which of the following precautions should be taken to prevent damage to the cannula:

a, b, d

a. Do not cut dressings that are around the cannula.

b. Do not puncture with a needle.

c. To clamp the tubing, use a clamp with teeth.

d. To clamp the tubing, use a clamp with a smooth surface—no teeth or ridges.

## Frame 5

The flow of the blood in a cannula is from the arterial tip to the venous tip. If you listen over the tubing with a stethoscope you should hear the turbulence of the arterial blood flow. This is called a *bruit*. The pulsation of this blood flow can also be palpated in the cannula or beyond the venous tip. This is called the *thrill*. The presence of a bruit or thrill indicates that the cannula is patent.

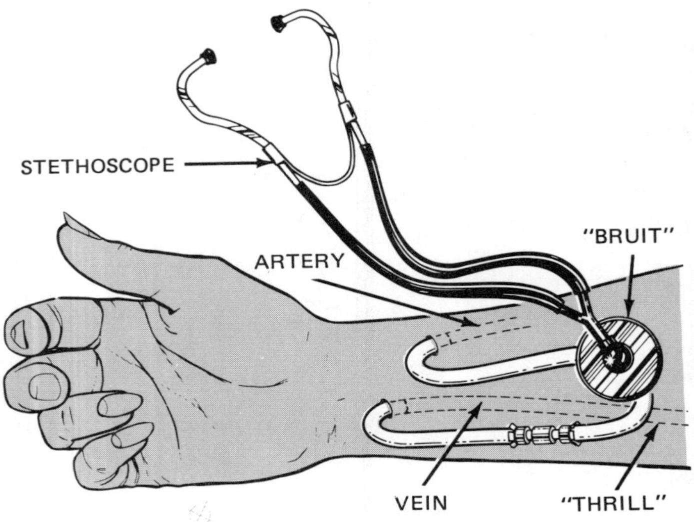


Figure 53

1. Indicate with arrows, the direction of the blood flow in the cannula in this figure.
2. The sound of the blood flow is the (bruit/thrill).
3. The thrill is (heard/palpated).
4. If the cannula is patent the bruit or thrill is (absent/present).
5. Blood in the cannula is (arterial/venous).

1. from artery to vein
2. bruit
3. palpated
4. present
5. arterial

## Frame 6

A patient with a new cannula should be observed closely for postoperative complications every 15 minutes for the first hour.

A cannulation procedure will normally cause some incisional discomfort and bleeding. There may be swelling around the exit sites and of the hand or foot. A cannulation interrupts the normal blood supply. Therefore, the patient may have numbness and tingling of the affected hand or foot. This should stop when collateral circulation develops. Numbness, due to nerve damage, may last several months or be permanent.

Incisional aching will probably begin as the local anesthetic wears off. It should be relieved by an analgesic. Unrelieved or severe pain due to vessel spasms should be reported to the doctor. Bleeding on inside dressings is expected but should subside after the first day. Recall that uremic patients have abnormal platelet function that slows blood clotting. Blood-soaked dressings or continuous oozing to the outer dressings should be reported.

Elevating the extremity above heart level can help reduce the pain and bleeding and any swelling. If the edema continues to swell or extends to the arm or leg, it should be reported to the doctor.

Mr. Jamison had been in his room for 1 hour since the cannulation when he began to complain of incisional aching in the area of the cannula. In checking further, Ellen found 4 cm red blood on the inside dressings.

1. Are these findings unusual?

2. Choose the measures Ellen would initiate:

    a. Administer an analgesic.
    b. Cradle cannulated arm on two pillows.

1. no (Aching probably due to loss of anesthetic. Blood only on inside dressings.)

2. a, b, d (Mr. Jamison should be rechecked soon, perhaps every 15 min.)

c. Recheck Mr. Jamison in 4 hours.
d. Reassure Mr. Jamison that these are normal postoperative findings.

## Frame 7

Several hours after the cannulation, Mr. Jamison began complaining of cramping pains in his left arm. Ellen knew that painful vessel spasms can occur due to the irritation of the surgery and that clotting of the cannula would probably follow if the spasms continued. The doctor ordered a stronger analgesic and continuous warm moist packs. Ellen worked to keep the cannulated extremity (and Mr. Jamison) relaxed, quiet, and comfortable. Detection of further problems became a priority.

What measures are important when vessel spasms are present?

a, b, d, e

a. Report the pain to the doctor.
b. Administer medication.
c. Apply cold packs.
d. Apply warm, moist packs.
e. Increase frequency of observation.

## Frame 8

The blood in a patent cannula is the red of fresh arterial blood and it warms the tubing to body temperature. The blood flow turbulence can be heard and palpated.

Clotting is a frequent complication even with the special plastics used to make the cannulas. It may occur anytime, but causative factors include

- Venous spasm due to vessel trauma during surgery
- Infection of the vessel
- Hypotension causing a decreased blood flow
- Sleeping on the cannulated extremity
- Excessive, vigorous use of the extremity.

It is important to know what to look for in checking for a clotted cannula. As the blood clots it turns dark and may separate into layers of plasma and cells. The cannula will feel cooler than body temperature. On auscultation, no blood flow turbulence is heard.

Choose the signs and symptoms of a clotted cannula:

b, c, e

a. The cannula is warm to the touch.
b. The cannula is cold to the touch.
c. The red cells are a very dark red.
d. The blood is bright red.
e. There are two layers in the blood tubing.
f. A loud bruit may be heard.

**Frame 9**

As Ellen checked the cannula she noticed it had turned darker and she could no longer hear a bruit.

The clotting complication most often involves only the shunt and is therefore not considered a medical emergency. To preserve the cannula's use it should be declotted as soon as possible by trained personnel. Declotting is usually done by trying to remove the clotted blood by aspirating and irrigating with a solution of heparinized saline.

Since Mr. Jamison's cannula was cool, with dark red blood in the tubing, what should Ellen do first?

a. Irrigate the cannula with 25 ml normal saline.
b. Clamp the cannula.
c. Notify dialysis personnel—physician and/or nurse.

c. (It may not be necessary to clamp the already clotted cannula.)

The dialysis personnel decided to declot the cannula as soon as Mr. Jamison could be brought to the dialysis unit.

## Frame 10

Several days later, when Mr. Jamison's abdominal wound bleeding had stopped, he was begun on systemic anticoagulation with warfarin (Coumadin). This was to help prevent further cannula clotting.

Since patients with renal disease already bleed easily, which of these symptoms should Ellen observe for in Mr. Jamison?

g.

a. Bruises
b. Nose bleeds
c. Tarry stools
d. Hematemesis
e. Bleeding gums
f. Incisional hemorrhage
g. All of the above

## Frame 11

Infection is another common problem of the external access. The increased incidences may be due to the nonadherence of the skin around the tubing (exit sites) and to the frequent opening of the cannula for dialysis. Both allow direct pathways for introduction of pathogens.

The first signs of infection usually appear around the exit sites. They may be painful, reddened and swollen. There may be drainage that is purulent, serous or bloody.

Select symptoms Ellen looked for in observing a cannula for infection.

a, c, d, f

a. Unusual drainage or bleeding around exit sites
b. Cyanosis of the fingernails
c. Tenderness
d. Reddened skin
e. Atrophy of arm muscles
f. Unusual swelling around the exit sites

Cultures of drainage are taken and antibiotic therapy is begun early. A severly infected cannula may be removed before systemic infection begins. Removal of the infected cannula means loss of a dialysis access site. Keeping the cannula clean is one way of preventing infection.

*Panel 2*

*It is important to keep a cannula clean and dry to prevent infection and trauma. Ellen changed Mr. Jamison's dressing on the days he did not dialyze. She used aseptic technique to protect the cannula and she wore gloves to protect herself from the risk of hepatitis. She did not use a scissors to remove the old dressings, to avoid accidental cutting of the tubing. She also used care not to pull or tug the cannula. Unnecessary movement of the cannula may cause problems that will decrease the time the shunt can be used.*

*Ellen's procedure for cleansing the shunt included applying hydrogen peroxide around the exit sites and then removing loosened matter. Next, she applied an antiseptic solution around the sites. She wiped off the Silastic tubing with an antiseptic sponge and washed Mr. Jamison's arm under the dressing area. On dialysis days a similar cleansing was done before and after the procedure.*

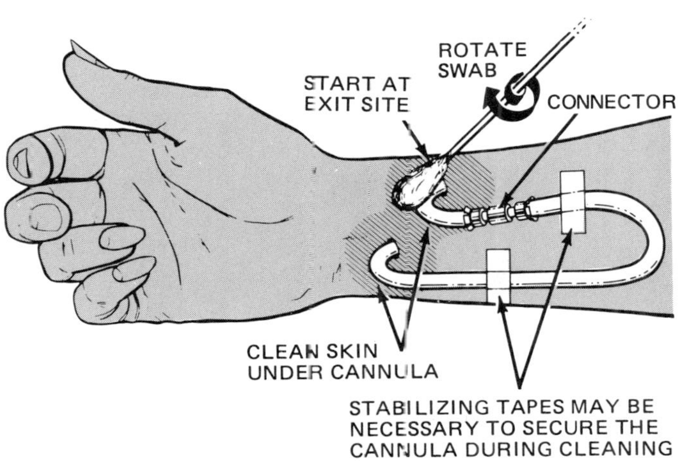


Figure 54

*As she cleansed the cannula, she inspected it for signs of infection and clotting. She also checked the connector for a correct fit and assured that the cannula was lying properly so it would not be kinked.*

*Ellen wrapped the entire cannula in a layer of gauze for protection. She could easily pull down the top portion to check for evidence of clotting.*

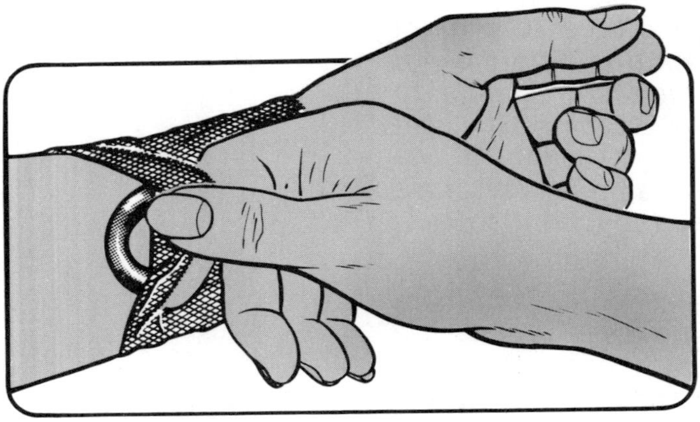

Figure 55

*The last thing Ellen did was to replace the smooth cannula clamps. These clamps are worn by the patient at all times. In case of an accidental separation the ends of the cannula can be clamped to stop the hemorrhage.*

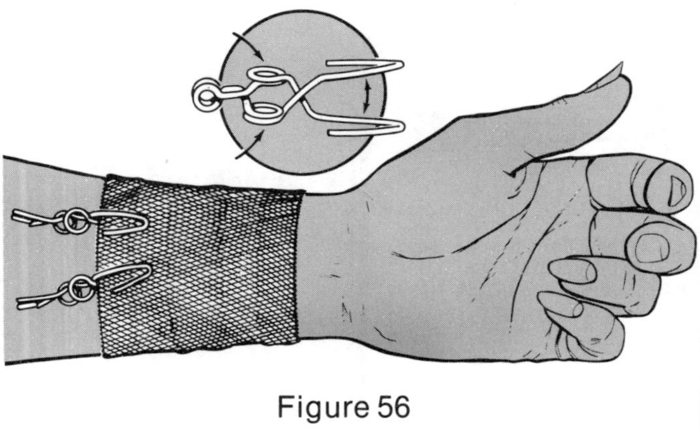

Figure 56

*If a cannula end comes out of its exit site, direct pressure with the heel of the hand must be applied to the site. The attached tubing must be clamped off.*

*When Mr. Jamison was able to bathe and shower, his cannula dressings were kept dry with a plastic wrap. Wet dressings were changed immediately.*

Refer to Panel 2 for Frames 12, 13, and 14.

**Frame 12**

How did Ellen accomplish the following objectives when she cleansed Mr. Jamison's cannula?

a. Removal of organic matter

b. Reduction in number of bacteria

a. Applied hydrogen peroxide. Removed loosened matter

b. Applied an antiseptic. Wiped Silastic tubing with an antiseptic

**Frame 13**

Match the measures Ellen used while cleaning the cannula to their purpose:

a. To prevent infection
b. To prevent clotting

1. ______ Thorough handwashing before beginning
2. ______ No unnecessary tugging or pulling
3. ______ Stabilizing tapes kept in place
4. ______ Cleansing with an antiseptic
5. ______ Checking for kinks
6. ______ Wrapping the cannula in a sterile dressing
7. ______ Upper part of dressing could be easily pulled down
8. ______ Plastic wrap of dressing during bath

1. a
2. b (also a)
3. b (also a)
4. a
5. b
6. a
7. b
8. a

## Frame 14

What did Ellen do during cannula care to protect herself against hepatitis?

She wore gloves. (Masks may also be required at some hospitals)

Hepatitis will be discussed at the end of this chapter.

## Frame 15

1. List the two common complications of an external access:
2. What are the symptoms of each?

1. Infection
   Clotting
2. Infection: redness, tenderness, pain, swelling, unusual bleeding or drainage

   Clotting: absence of a bruit and thrill, cooling of cannula temperature, darkening and separation of blood in cannula

## Frame 16

Another possible complication of an external shunt is separation with hemorrhage.

Mr. Melby is your dialysis patient. Suddenly you hear him yelling, "Nurse, Nurse! Somebody help me!" You find him pinching both ends of the cannula in his left arm with his right fingers. The cannula has come apart and in spite of his squeezing, he's still losing blood.

1. What should you do?
   a. Panic!
   b. Manually squeeze the tubing until you can get the clamps on.

1. b, d

c. Grab any available object that could clamp off the tubing.
d. Use only smooth cannula clamps.

2. What should you do if a cannula end had fallen out?

2. Apply direct pressure to the site with the heel of your hand. Clamp off the attached tubing.

Other external shunt complications include phlebitis due to irritation of the vessel and erosion of the shunt tips through the overlying skin.

**Frame 17**

Summary:
There are two main categories of hemodialysis access: internal and external. If possible, they are created in the nondominant arm.

*External Access*

The Shaldon catheter is a temporary access that can be placed in the femoral vein. A permanent access is called a shunt or cannula. Tubing is placed in an artery and a vein, with a connector that opens for attachment to the machine. Types of shunts are: Scribner, Buselmeier, and Thomas Femoral.

Clotting and infection are the two major access complications. Infection is recognized by redness, tenderness, swelling, and unusual bleeding or drainage. Clotting of an external access can be noted by a cooling in cannula temperature, darkening and separating of the blood, and absence of a bruit.

Advantages and Disadvantages

The external access is readily put in place and a venipuncture is not required for dialysis. Since it is more susceptible to infection and clotting, it is not able to be used for long periods of time. The person having one has restricted movement of the extremity and needs to change the dressing daily.

## Internal Type

An internal access is developed by joining an adjacent artery and vein, either directly or with a graft.

Suzanne Rice had a simple fistula developing for future use with hemodialysis. This is one kind of internal access.

*Panel 3*
*The simple fistula is created by anastomosis of a vein and an artery. After a local anesthetic, an incision is made, usually at the wrist, to locate the appropriate vein and artery.*

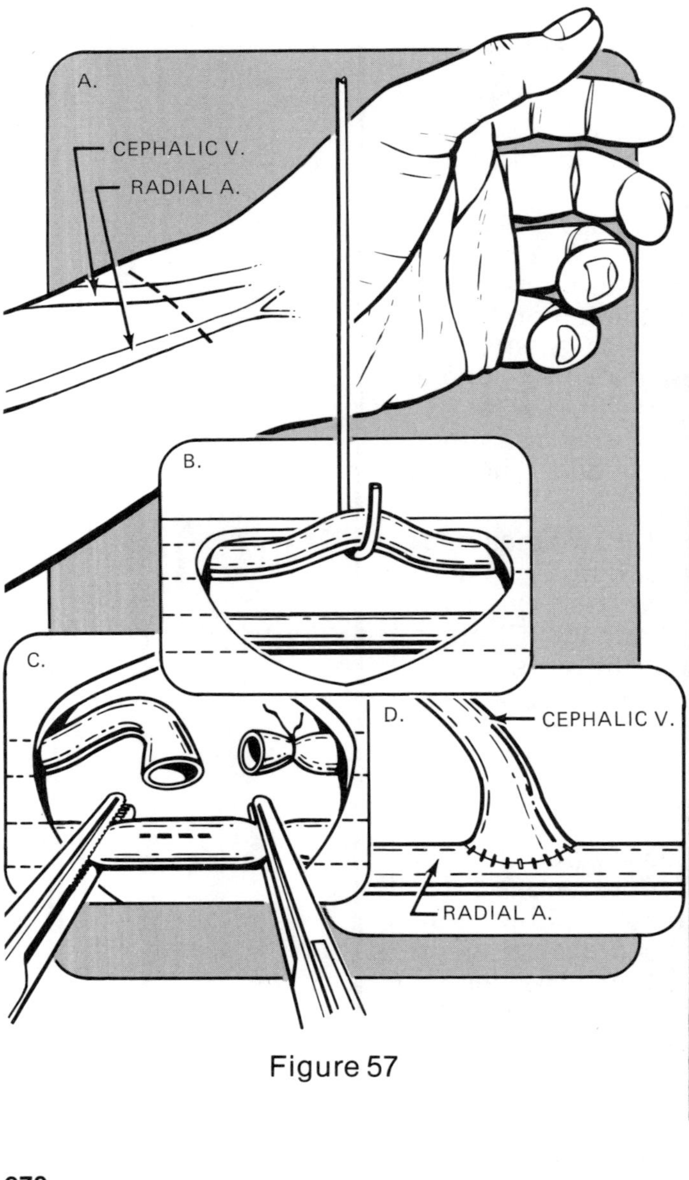


Figure 57

*The vein and artery may be anastomosed in several ways: 1) end to end, 2) artery end to vein side, 3) vein end to artery side or 4) side to side. After the blood flow through the fistula has been evaluated, the incision is closed. (Arrows indicate direction of blood flow.)*

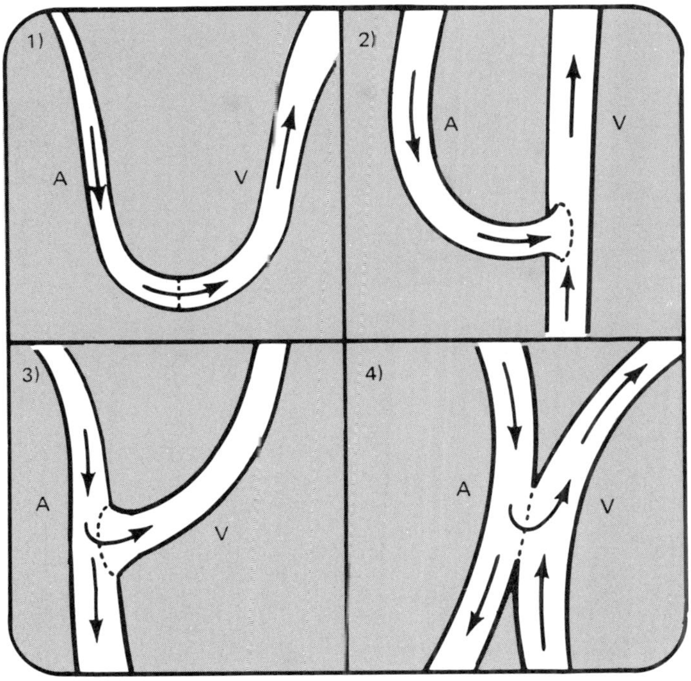


Figure 58

*The anastomosis or fistula allows the development of an* arterialized *vein, or fistula vein. This vein enlarges, "matures," and develops a stronger blood flow rate. The vein can then be used for hemodialysis as it will tolerate repeated venipuncture with needles of large diameter and will provide a good flow of arterial blood for hemodialysis.*

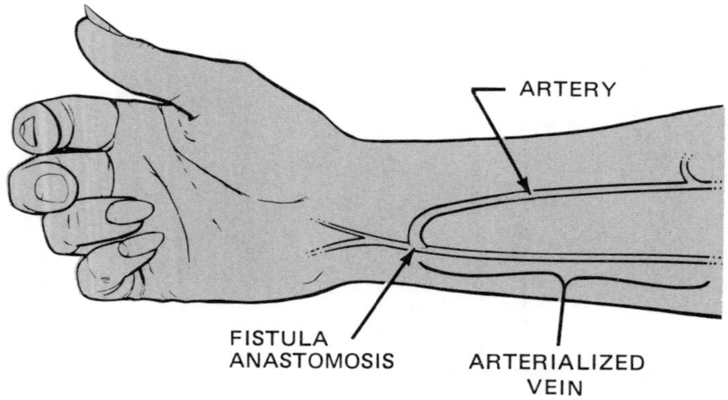


Figure 59

*Bovine graft*

*A carotid artery from a cow is cleaned and treated to remove antigenic properties. The tube that remains is then suitable for use as a graft. It is sutured into place as pictured below. The body of the graft is tunneled under the skin to form a U-shape. The Bovine graft ends are anastomosed to incisions in a vein and an artery near the antecubital fossa.*
*The blood vessels can also be joined by using a graft.*

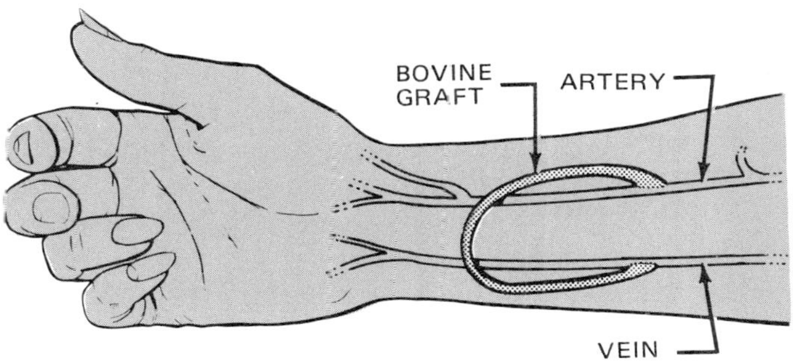


Figure 60

*Man-made materials:*

*A type of Dacron graft is sutured in place. During the maturing period, the patients endothelium and epithelium grow around the graft. It is then used as an access site.*

*Homograft*

*Part of the patient's saphenous vein can be used as a graft.*

## Frame 18

The postop observation of a simple fistula is similar to that of a new cannula. Can you recall five or six observations that apply to both? (Hint: see Frames 5 and 6.)

Check for
1. patency—presence of a bruit
2. amount of bleeding
3. level of pain
4. numbness
5. tingling
6. swelling

The graft fistulas cause greater swelling than the simple fistula or cannula. It may be similar to that seen with mastectomies. The patient's arm needs to be elevated 3–5 days. The amount of elevation required may be accomplished by extending the arm toward the ceiling. This could be done by tying it to an IV pole. Patients who have grafts usually have more bleeding, pain, and numbness than patients with other types of access.

## Frame 19

The pressure from the arterial blood flowing through the simple fistula vein causes it to enlarge. As the diameter increases the wall becomes thicker. A bruit is present because of blood flow turbulence. The fistula vein is also referred to as an "arterialized vein."

1. The blood flowing through the simple fistula is (arterial/venous).
2. The absence of a bruit probably means the fistula (is/is not) patent.

1. arterial
2. is not

A simple fistula vein enlarges due to the increased blood flow but to withstand the repetitive venipunctures it must also toughen or "mature." Most surgeons recommend some type of fistula-maturing exercise. An example is asking the patient to clench and unclench his fist while the vein is occluded by a tourniquet. The exercise routine begins several days postop and continues until the vessel can be used for dialysis.

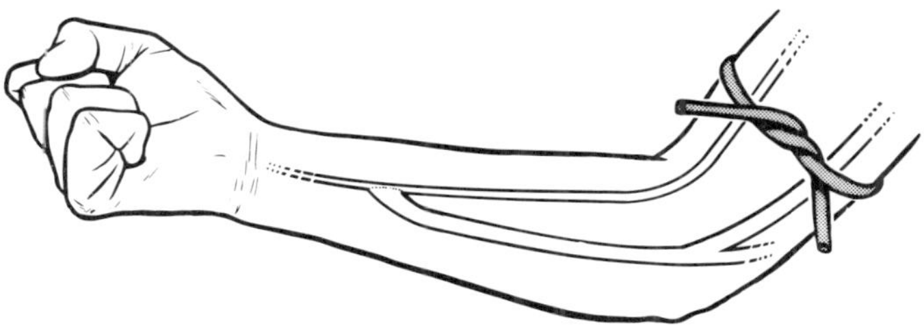

Figure 61

## Frame 20

The fistula needles used for dialysis are labeled arterial and venous.

Arterial needle: Blood passes *from* the patient into the dialysis system.

Venous needle: Blood returns *to* the patient after purification in the dialyzer.

This figure shows an example of where the needles may be placed for dialysis.

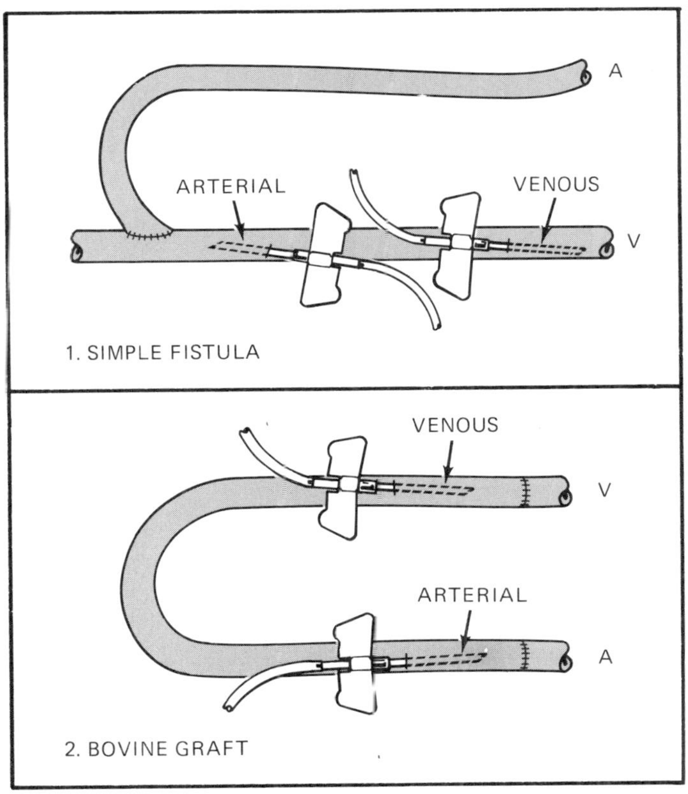


Figure 62

1. In these examples the arterial needle points (away from/toward) the artery to better receive the flow of blood.

   1. toward

2. The venous needle points toward a (vein/artery).

   2. vein

3. The blood returning in the venous needle has had exchanges of ($K/CO_2/Na$).

   3. K, Na

4. As the arterialized vein of the simple fistula is used during dialysis, (arterial/venous) blood is flowing in it.

   4. arterial

*Panel 4*

*Here are the advantages and disadvantages of a fistula:*

| Advantages | Disadvantages |
|---|---|
| *Can be used over a long time period (several months to several years)* | *Must settle in or mature before it can be used (2–8 weeks depending on type)* |
| *Less restrictions in use of the access extremity* | *Requires two venipunctures for each dialysis (A one-needle system has been tried but more hours of dialysis are then needed.)* |
| *Less incidences of clotting or infection* | |
| *Simple to care for as there is no opening to the skin surface* | |

**Frame 21**

Infection and clotting are also fistula complications.

1. What signs and symptoms would indicate infection?
   a. A mature fistula that is very tender
   b. Unusual redness
   c. Swelling over puncture sites
   d. Drainage
   e. Absence of a bruit

   1. a, b, c, d

2. Which of the above signs and symptoms could indicate a clotted fistula?

   2. a, e (possibly c)

Other fistula complications include failure to develop, hemorrhage from puncture sites, aneurysm, and ischemia of the hand ("steal syndrome").

## Frame 22

Referring to the figure, fill in the blanks to complete the following statements:

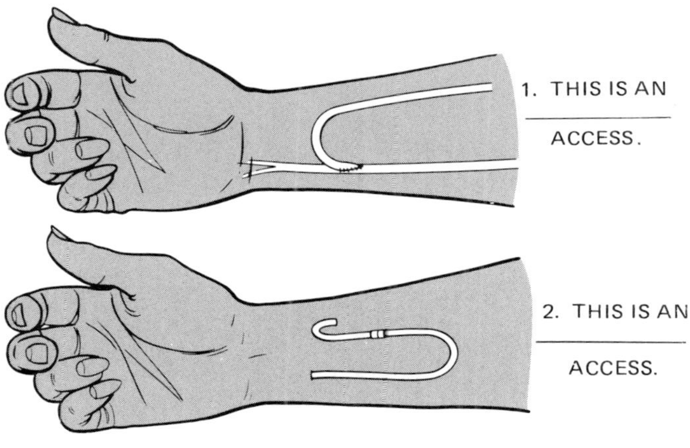


Figure 63

1. internal (simple fistula)

2. external (cannula)

## Frame 23

Decide if the following phrases apply to an internal or external access:

a. ____________ Entirely under the skin

b. ____________ An appliance sewn into a blood vessel with an extension outside the skin

c. ____________ Requires a special shunt connector for hookup to the dialyzer

d. ____________ Requires venipuncture with a large gauge needle for hookup to the dialyzer

a. Internal

b. External

c. External

d. Internal

## Frame 24

Mark the following statements true or false:

1. ______ One cannula can be used for several years.
2. ______ Fistulas require venipunctures for dialysis.
3. ______ A cannula is more prone to infection than a fistula.
4. ______ A fistula is more prone to clotting than a cannula.
5. ______ A simple fistula can be used immediately after creation.

1. False
2. True
3. True
4. False
5. False

## Frame 25

Blood vessels needed for hemodialysis should be preserved from trauma.

Referring to the figure, fill in the blanks to complete the following statement:

Do not ______________ or ______________ from an extremity with either an external or internal access site.

take a blood pressure

draw blood or inject an IV medication

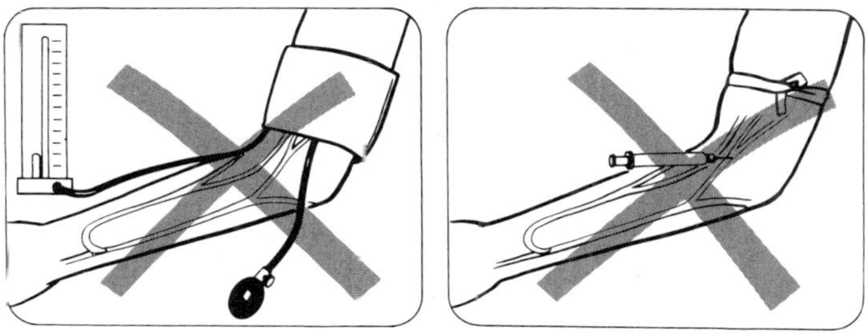

Figure 64

## Frame 26

Summary:

*Internal Access*

An internal access is created by surgically joining an adjacent artery and vein or by implanting a graft that joins these vessels.

Advantages and Disadvantages

An internal access is preferred when there is time for it to mature before use. It is less susceptible to infection and to clotting problems and can be used for a longer time than external access. Because an internal access is all under the skin it is easier to care for and most patients do not mind the necessary venipunctures for dialysis.

Names of internal access are: simple AV fistula, Bovine graft, Vortex graft, and saphenous vein graft.

# PART III PROCEDURE

Mr. Jamison is in the dialysis unit waiting to be connected to a dialyzer. You are going to find out how this procedure is carried out. You already know some important things about making dialysis possible.

## Frame 27

You've looked at several types of access used to connect people to the dialysis system. Fill in the blanks to complete the statements.

1. A Scribner shunt (cannula) is an example of an ___________ access.
2. A simple AV fistula is an example of an ___________ shunt.

1. external
2. internal

## Frame 28

You've learned the three components that must come in contact for dialysis to occur.

Choose the three components:

a. The patient's blood
b. A nonpermeable membrane
c. Blood transfusions
d. A semipermeable membrane
e. Dialysate

a, d, e

## Frame 29

You have also studied what normal-kidney functions are carried out by the artificial kidney. Select them from the following:

a. Removal of excess fluid
b. Removal of metabolic waste
c. Restoration of electrolyte levels
d. Removal of protein
e. Restoration of acid-base balance

a, b, c, e

*Panel 5*

*Before beginning dialysis, Mr. Jamison is weighed, and his blood pressure, pulse and respiratory rates, and temperature are measured. Mr. Jamison is being dialyzed in a hospital bed.*

*Anne, the nurse in the dialysis unit, clamps off Mr. Jamison's cannula. She then removes the connector piece replacing it with special adaptors enabling hookup to the tubing leading to and from the dialyzer.*

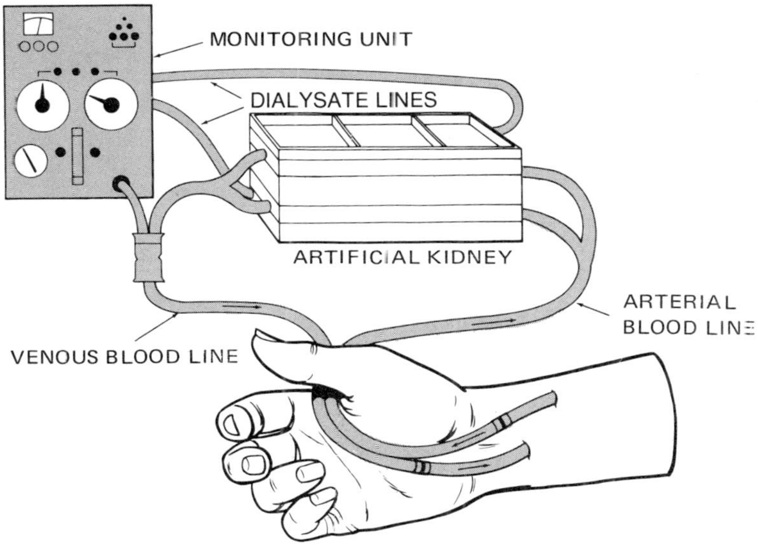


Figure 65

*When the clamps are removed, the pumping action of Mr. Jamison's heart begins to move his blood into the dialyzer.*

*Because Mr. Jamison has had problems with hypotension and hypovolemia due to blood loss, the dialyzer's blood compartments have been filled with normal saline. This is infused into Mr. Jamison through the venous connection and prevents hypotension as his blood fills the dialyzer. This is called a* prime.

*As the process of dialysis begins, the blood pump is turned on. As shown in the following figure, the blood pump is located on the arterial blood line. Its purpose is to help the heart propel the blood through the dialyzer at a constant rate.*

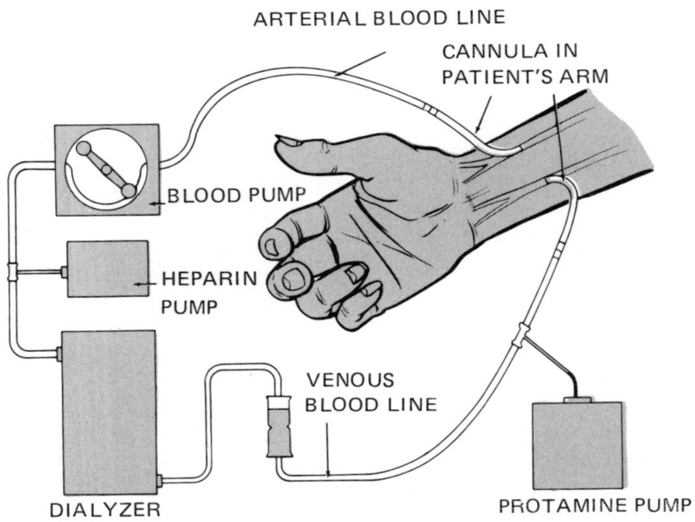


Figure 66

*To keep Mr. Jamison's blood from clotting in the dialyzer, a constant infusion of heparin is added to the arterial blood. Find the heparin infusion pump in the figure.*

*Because Mr. Jamison has recently had surgery, the heparin effect must be counteracted before his blood returns to him. Protamine is infused into the venous blood line to prevent systemic heparinization.*

*Now that Anne has Mr. Jamison on dialysis, she will recheck his vital signs (blood pressure, pulse, respiration).*

## Frame 30

Match these features of dialysis with their description and/or reason for use:

1. ___ Blood pump
2. ___ Prime
3. ___ Heparin
4. ___ Protamine
5. ___ Cannula
6. ___ Arterial blood line
7. ___ Venous blood line

a. Tubing that returns the patient's blood from the dialyzer
b. Prevents blood clotting in the dialyzer
c. Connection point between patient and dialyzer
d. Tubing that brings the patient's blood to the dialyzer
e. Prevents systemic heparinization
f. Assists the heart to propel blood into the dialyzer
g. Filling of blood compartments with saline before dialysis to prevent hypotension

1. f
2. g
3. b
4. e
5. c
6. d
7. a

## Frame 31

Recall from Panel 5 that an infusion of heparin is used to keep the blood from clotting in the dialyzer. There are several ways to do this. *Systemic* heparinization (both patient and dialyzer) is accomplished by infusing an average of 1,000–1,500 U/hour into the arterial blood line. If the patient should not be anticoagulated, a *regional* technique is used; the dialyzer is anticoagulated in the usual manner, but protamine is infused into the venous return, keeping the patient at a normal clotting time.

1. Mr. Jamison received both heparin and protamine infusions. This is what type of heparinization?
2. Why did Mr. Jamison require regional heparinization?

1. Regional
2. Recent surgery increased risk of bleeding.

## Frame 32

The dialyzer or artificial kidney is the most obvious piece of equipment needed for hemodialysis. Most dialyzers are made of four basic components:

Dialyzing fluid compartment
Blood compartment
Semipermeable membrane
Membrane support structure

You've looked at the first three components. The support structure keeps the compartments separated. The hemodialyzer membranes are either a tube, sheet or spun hollow fiber of cellulose.

What do you recall about the permeability of these membranes? (Hint: see Chapter 12, Panel 1).

They're semi-permeable to small molecules, electrolytes, water, glucose, and metabolic waste. They're impermeable to large molecules, blood cells, protein, and bacteria.

*Panel 6*

A. THE COIL DIALYZER

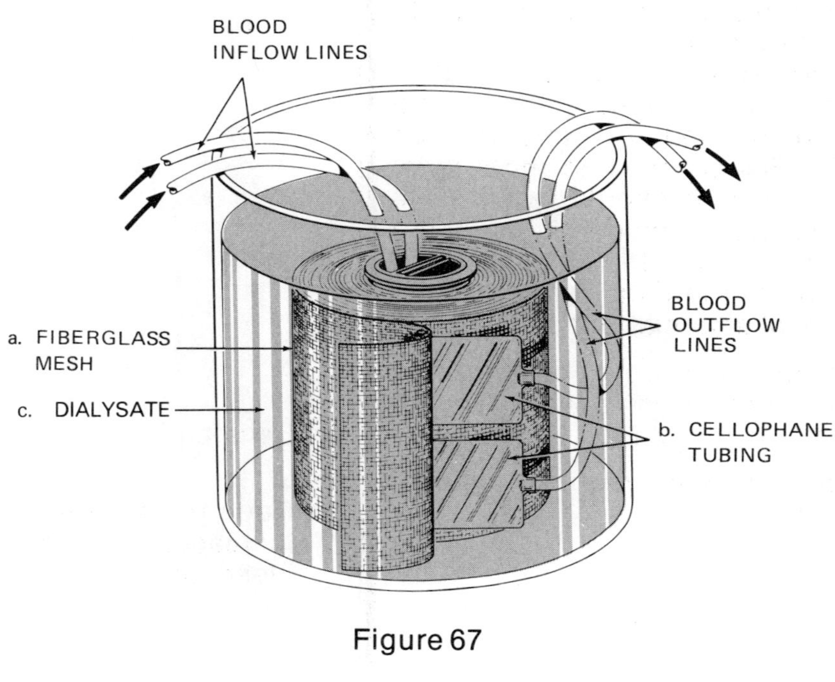


Figure 67

*Panel 6*, continued

*The coil dialyzer contains one or two long tubes of cellulose membrane (b), supported by a rigid plastic mesh (a). Blood is pumped into the cellulose tube which is rolled up jelly-roll fashion. The coil is submerged in a "pot" of dialysate (c). The dialysate freely circulates around the coiled membrane through the open mesh support structure.*

B. THE FLAT PLATE DIALYSER

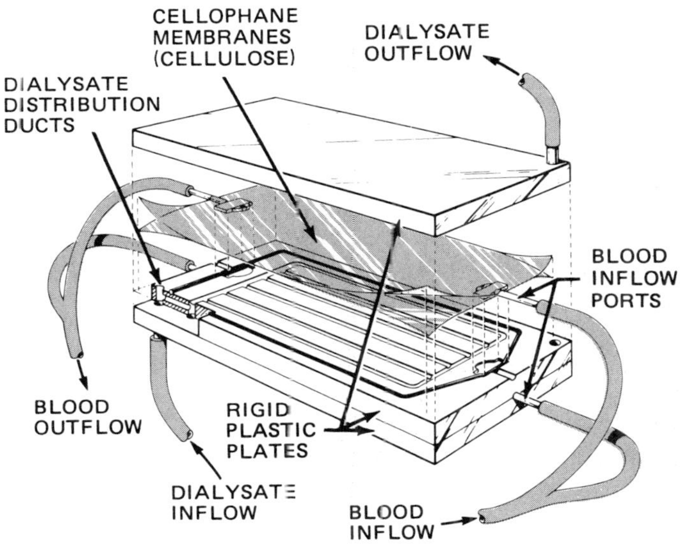


Figure 68

*The flat-plate dialyzer contains sheets of cellulose sandwiched between rigid polypropylene plates. Blood is pumped into envelopes of cellulose membrane. Dialysate is pumped into the space between the blood layers.*

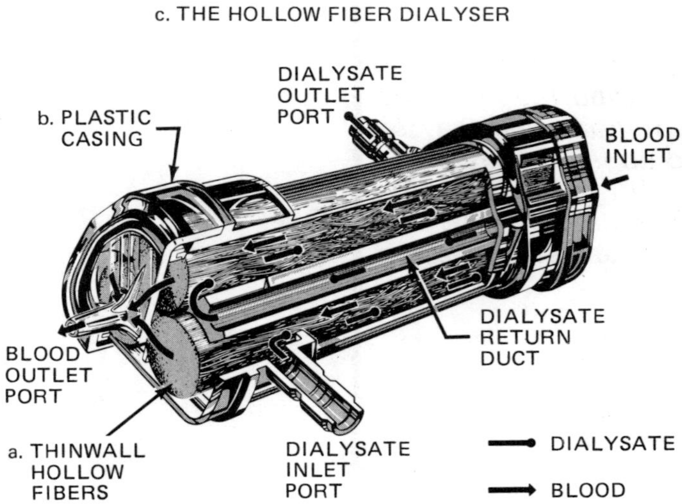


Figure 69

*The hollow-fiber dialyzer stemmed from the development of a method of spinning cellulose acetate into tiny hollow fibers. Thousands of fibers (a) are encased in a clear plastic case—about the size of a large flashlight (b). Blood is pumped into the hollow fibers and dialysate is pumped around the outside of the fibers, which constitute the membrane.*

## Frame 33

Mark the following statements true or false:

1. ______ Blood and dialysate mix freely in one large compartment.

2. ______ All dialyzers have four major components.

3. ______ There are three basic types of artificial kidneys, which all work on the same principles.

Recall that the three physical processes used in dialysis are diffusion for solute balance and osmosis and filtration to remove water.

1. False (Blood and dialysate have their own compartments and are separated by the cellulose membrane.)
2. True
3. True

*Panel 7*

*Filtration is a process of fluid removal that is helped by gravity. Since this can be a slow process, the rate of fluid removal in hemodialysis is increased by* ultrafiltration.

*Methods of Ultrafiltration*

1. *Positive pressure on the blood compartment*

   *Water flows from an area of high pressure to an area of lower pressure. Fluid from the blood will move more rapidly through the semipermeable membrane if pressure is increased in the blood compartment.*

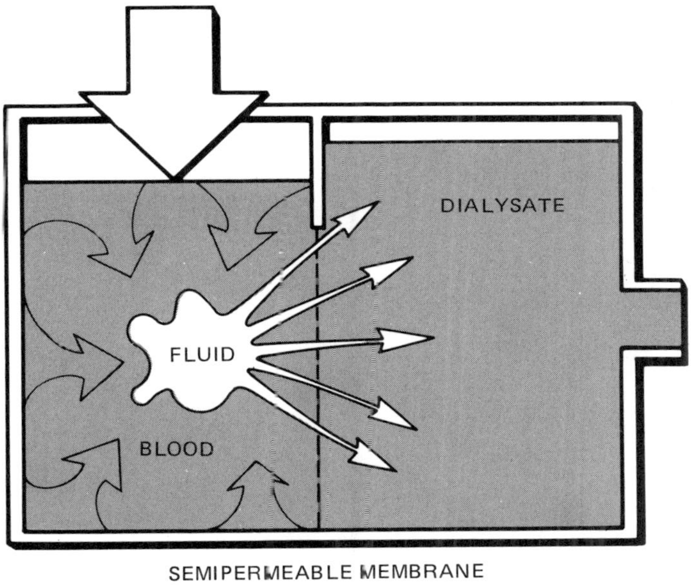


Figure 70

2. *Negative pressure on the dialysate compartment.*

   *This uses the same principle. By creating a vacuum in the dialysis compartment, more fluid is pulled through the semipermeable membrane.*

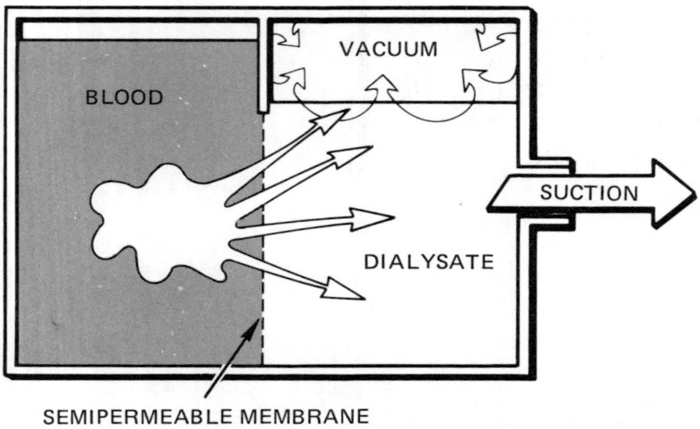


Figure 71

## Frame 34

Mr. Jamison is being dialyzed with a flat-plate dialyzer with ultrafiltration. Negative pressure is the method being used to remove fluid.

Mark these statements true or false:

1. ______ Ultrafiltration will accelerate the removal of excess fluid.

2. ______ Negative pressure is being put on the blood compartment.

1. True

2. False

## Frame 35

Osmosis may also be employed during hemodialysis. The glucose concentration in dialysate is higher than in the blood. This would cause water to move out of the ____________ and into the ____________.

blood
dialysate

## Frame 36

Acid-base and electrolyte balance are regulated by adding various amounts of solutes to dialysis. Metabolic waste is also cleared by the process of diffusion.

Mr. Jamison's serum potassium level is 6 mEq. The dialysate has 3 mEq potassium. Which way would potassium diffuse?

Into the dialysate

*Panel 8*

*Special precautions are required to make hemodialysis a safe procedure. A system is provided to prepare, deliver, and monitor an accurately warmed and proportioned dialysate. The venous blood line is monitored for changes in blood flow resistance and the presence of air. Begin at #1 in the figure for a "tour" of these systems.*

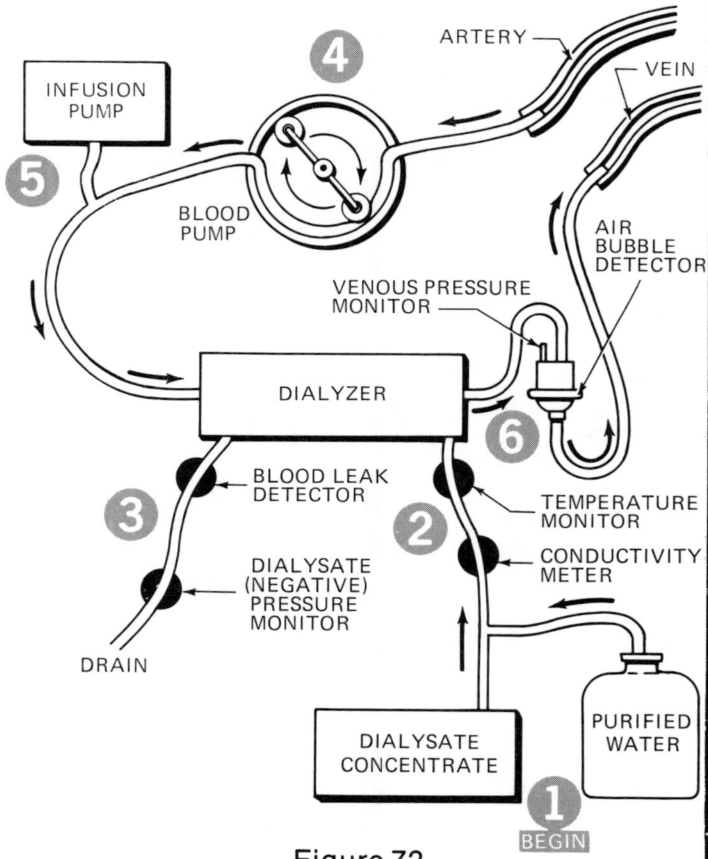


Figure 72

### Dialysate compartment

1. *Purified water combines with a dialysate solution and goes into the machine. Water need not be sterile, as bacteria do not cross the hemodialysis membrane. The water is softened, filtered or de-ionized to remove such substances as nitrates, sulfates, and other unwanted solutes.*
2. *The conductivity monitor tests dialysate composition by measuring the ions' electric charge.*

   *The temperature of the dialysate is important. If the patient's blood is too warm, hemolysis may occur; if too cold, the patient will have chilling.*
3. *The blood leak detector will detect any blood escaping from the blood compartments into the dialysate. The negative pressure monitor keeps ultrafiltration within safe limits, so too much fluid is not withdrawn.*

### Blood compartment

4. *Blood flows from the patient's artery, and its flow through the machine is aided by the blood pump.*
5. *The infusion pump is used to add heparin to the blood.*
6. *After blood flows through the machine, it returns to the patient through the venous blood line. The venous pressure monitor senses changes in the blood pressure. This could be from a clot or a kink in the tubing, a sudden drop in the patient's blood pressure, or blood line separation. The air bubble detector prevents the infusion of air into the patient's vascular system.*

## Frame 37

Match each problem situation with the monitor that should detect it.

| | | |
|---|---|---|
| 1. ______ Torn membrane allowing blood to leak into the dialysate | a. Air bubble detector | 1. b |
| 2. ______ Too little negative pressure for ultrafiltration | b. Blood leak detector | 2. f |
| 3. ______ Dialysate too warm or too cold | c. Venous pressure monitor | 3. e |
| 4. ______ Blood pump sucking in air due to a loose arterial cannula connection | d. Conductivity meter (dialysate composition) | 4. a |
| 5. ______ Systemic hypotension due to removal of too much fluid from the blood | e. Dialysate temperature monitor | 5. c |
| 6. ______ Hypotonic or hypertonic dialysate | f. Dialysate pressure monitor | 6. d |

## Frame 38

Anne has answered a monitor alarm on Mr. Jamison's dialyzer. He had turned over and kinked off the venous tubing.

1. Was the dialysate or venous pressure monitor alerted?
2. Why?

1. venous
2. The kinked venous tubing created a resistance which increased the pressure inside the tubing.

One day Mr. Jamison spiked a high temperature during dialysis. The doctors said it was a "pyrogen reaction." A pyrogen is a substance produced by bacteria. This will cross the membrane and the body treats it as any invading foreign substance.

After Mr. Jamison has dialyzed 6 hours, Anne will take him off dialysis. To do this she will turn off the infusion and blood pumps. The arterial connection will be clamped off and all of Mr. Jamison's blood returned to him. The cannula ends are then joined by a sterile connector.

Before returning to his room, Mr. Jamison will be weighed to see how much fluid was lost and his blood pressure, pulse, respiration, and temperature will be checked for evidence of hypotension or a febrile response.

## Frame 39

Summary:

There are three basic types of dialyzers presently in use. They are the coil, flat-plate, and hollow-fiber. All dialyzers have four components which are *1)* a blood compartment, and *2)* a dialysate compartment separated by *3)* a semipermeable membrane which has *4)* a support structure.

Several extra pieces of equipment and monitors are used to make hemodialysis safer and more efficient. A blood pump may help move the blood through the dialyzer at about 225 ml/min. An infusion pump may add heparin or protamine. The blood line is checked for changes in pressure and for air bubbles. The dialysate solution is checked for accurate temperature and ion concentration, for presence of blood and for correct negative pressure.

## Physical Problems of Hemodialysis

## Frame 40

Some days when Mr. Jamison is in dialysis, he becomes hypovolemic and his blood pressure drops.

1. Can removal of too much fluid during dialysis cause hypovolemia?

   1. Yes

2. Select symptoms Mr. Jamison might have as his blood pressure drops:

   a, b, c, d, e, f

   a. Nausea
   b. Vomiting
   c. Light headedness
   d. Feeling of fainting
   e. Ringing in ears
   f. Anxiety
   g. Slow pulse

If this occurs, the dialysis nurse will turn off any negative pressure (suction) removing fluid. The patient will be put into a Trendelenburg position and a volume expander such as Ringers lactate or plasma will be infused rapidly.

Some patients who are on antihypertensive medications may have hypotension during dialysis due to the time of peak effect of the medication. In some cases hypotensives are not given before dialysis.

## Frame 41

Muscle cramps, usually in the form of severe spasms in the lower extremities, can occur during dialysis due to sodium and fluid shifts and losses.

Select the measures the nurse could use to help the patient be more comfortable: d

a. Help the patient work his or her feet against a foot board or the nurse's hands.

b. Help the patient stand and exercise his leg, if condition permits.

c. Apply warm packs to the affected area.

d. All of the above.

The dialysis nurse may also reduce the ultrafiltration pressure and thereby relieve the loss of sodium and fluid.

## Frame 42

A disequilibrium syndrome causes problems for some people going on dialysis.

Substances such as urea dialyze rapidly from the blood and then diffuse more slowly from the brain to the blood. The high levels of urea in the brain cause an osmotic pull of fluid to equalize the concentration.

Choose the symptoms you would expect with cerebral edema a, b, c, e, f, g

a. Headaches
b. Nausea
c. Vomiting
d. Chest pain
e. Confusion
f. Twitching
g. Seizures

# PART IV NURSING CARE OF PATIENTS FOLLOWING DIALYSIS

After Mr. Jamison's dialysis treatment he returned to the renal ICU. Ellen checked the dialysis report to find out if any of these situations occurred during the run:

Disequilibrium syndrome
Systemic heparinization
Hypovolemia due to ultrafiltration or a membrane leak of more than 500 ml blood
Elevated temperature

Each of these requires specific nursing interventions.

## Discussion

This response indicator consists of observations and interventions to be used following hemodialysis.

*Problem 1*

What nursing measures would help the patient who has disequilibrium syndrome? Squares numbered: ____________

*Problem 2*

Choose the nursing implications of systemic heparinization. Squares numbered: ____________

*Problem 3*

What should the nurse do if the patient became hypovolemic during dialysis? Squares numbered: ____________

*Problem 4*

What nursing actions are indicated for a problem with elevated temperature? Squares numbered: ____________

| Response Indicator | | | | |
|---|---|---|---|---|
| Take seizure precautions. 1 | Administer analgesics. 2 | Hold IM medications for 4 hours. 3 | Explain the cause of the problem to the patient. 4 | Increase frequency of monitoring blood pressure, temperature, pulse, and respiration. 5 |
| Administer antipyretic drugs. 6 | Explain safety measures for orthostatic hypotension to the patient. 7 | Prevent bumps, cuts, or other injury. 8 | Provide clear sensory cues to environment. 9 | Observe for signs of infection, especially lungs and access. 10 |
| Give cool sponge bath. 11 | Administer antiemetics. 12 | Observe for bleeding in stool, emesis, incision, and access. 13 | Do not administer drugs that primarily or secondarily lower blood pressure without asking physician. 14 | |

## Comments:

*Problem 1* — Disequilibrium Syndrome

Suggested responses: 1, 2, 4, 5, 9, 12.

Seizure precautions are wise. If the patient is confused, increase sensory cues: such as adequate lighting even at night, clearly marked bathroom doors, clearly visible clocks, calendars, and other items. The patient should know that this is a temporary problem. Analgesics and antiemetics can provide relief from symptoms, and a quiet atmosphere helps. It is good to keep close watch on the pulse, blood pressure, and other neuro signs.

*Problem 2* — Systemic Heparinization

Suggested responses: 3, 4, 8, 13.

The effects of the heparin infusion will last for about 4 hours. If possible, IM medications could be held to prevent bleeding within the muscle and subcutaneous tissue. The patient should be instructed to avoid bumps and bruises, and observations ought to be made for any untoward bleeding.

*Problem 3*— Hypovolemia

Suggested responses: 4, 5, 7, 14.

Careful observation of blood pressure and pulse are indicated until the body fluid compartments stabilize. This problem can be caused by excessive fluid loss and blood loss.

Find out about administering hypotensive drugs and instruct the patient to change position slowly and to call for assistance when getting out of bed.

*Problem 4* — Elevated Temperature

Suggested responses: 4, 5, 6, 10, 11.

Fever may be caused by a pyrogenic reaction or by underlying infection. So a close watch should be kept on the temperature and on signs of infection in vulnerable areas such as the respiratory system and access site. Antipyretic drugs and cool sponge baths will provide symptomatic relief.

## Frame 43

While caring for Mr. Jamison, Ellen continuously monitored the lab data and his weight to gauge the effectiveness of the daily dialysis treatments. Match the data with the renal function it monitors.

a. Fluid balance
b. Protein homeostasis
c. Solute equilibrium
d. Acid-base balance

| | | Answer |
|---|---|---|
| 1. ______ | Venous $CO_2$ content | 1. d |
| 2. ______ | Weight | 2. a |
| 3. ______ | BUN, creatinine | 3. c |
| 4. ______ | Blood pressure and pulse (supine and standing) | 4. a |
| 5. ______ | Arterial pH | 5. d |
| 6. ______ | Sodium, potassium | 6. c |
| 7. ______ | Serum albumin | 7. b |

## Frame 44

Today Mr. Jamison's potassium was 2.8 mEq when he returned from dialysis. Choose the action Ellen can take to help prevent any problems due to this:

a. Administer Kayexalate.
b. Give Mr. Jamison a food high in potassium such as raisins.

b

## Frame 45

Mr. Jamison had also had two episodes of hypotension during dialysis when fluid was being removed by ultrafiltration. He had gained 5 lb between dialysis treatments. A desirable weight gain between dialysis should be not greater than 1½ lb/day.

True or false:

1. ______ Ellen should review Mr. Jamison's intake patterns with him to decide how he can best stay within his fluid limits.
2. ______ One pound of weight gained is equivalent to 1,000 ml gained.

1. True
2. False (500 ml)

## Frame 46

The problem of hepatitis is fear provoking to patients, family, and staff members. After a week in the renal intensive care area, Mr. Jamison's wife began asking why so many of the patients were isolated. Ellen explained:

> Hepatitis is an inflammation of the liver due to a virus. We know there are two kinds of hepatitis-causing virus. Type A is transmitted by eating contaminated food. Type B is known to cross in blood transfusions and in body secretions. Type B is the hepatitis virus dialysis patients contact.
>
> We do everything we can to prevent Mr. Jamison and you from exposure to hepatitis. The dialyzers and tubing are all disposed of after each use. Needles are disposed of very carefully. Staff members wash their hands thoroughly when going between patients, and they wear gloves and masks

when opening blood lines. Patients who already have hepatitis are kept isolated from those who don't.

Blood transfusions are tested to be sure the virus is not present. And each month every dialysis patient's blood is tested to see if contact has been made with the virus.

If patients' blood shows they have contacted hepatitis virus, we let them know and teach them to initiate some isolation-type precautions to protect everyone. If staff members get hepatitis, they are not allowed to work until their doctors have determined it is safe.

Ellen's explanation helped Mrs. Jamison to understand the isolation policies of the renal ICU.

The risk of hepatitis is serious, and the outcome of the disease can be fatal. People can become chronic carriers even if there are no active symptoms. The best defense seems to be use of all preventative measures available, including

- Use of disposable equipment
- Isolation of patients with positive blood tests for hepatitis
- Thorough handwashing
- Use of gloves and masks when opening blood lines
- Protection of open wounds
- Safe disposal of needles
- No eating, drinking or smoking in the dialysis unit
- Cleansing of all flat surfaces with a Clorox solution
- Monthly screening for hepatitis $B_s$ antigen — all staff and patients

True or false:

1. ______ Hepatitis is caused by a virus.
2. ______ Type B virus is transmitted by contact with blood and body secretions.

1. True

2. True

3. ______ Adequate prevention of hepatitis transmission to staff members is achieved by the use of mask and glove techniques when caring for access sites and blood tubing.

3. False (Also needed are handwashing, environmental asepsis, isolation techniques, and careful disposal of used equipment.)

## Frame 47

Summary:

Advantages and disadvantages of Hemodialysis

Advantages

1. Efficient so less hours are spent dialyzing
2. Can provide a rapid change of fluid and chemical levels

Disadvantages

1. Special equipment and staff required
2. Fluid and chemical levels may be changed too rapidly
3. Heparinization required
4. Access complications can cause many problems
5. Blood transfusions may be needed

Physical Side Effects

The patient may experience symptoms due to fluid and solute changes during dialysis. Hypovolemia and/or hypotension may cause nausea, vomiting, light headedness, and anxiety. Muscle cramps may occur as sodium and fluid move. Symptoms of cerebral edema may occur if fluid is pulled into the brain to equalize the urea levels in the brain and the blood.

Summary (continued):

Nursing care following dialysis includes: follow-up observations and interventions appropriate to the complications mentioned. The patient should also be observed for changes in vital signs as stabilization occurs within the body. Signs of bleeding should be noted following systemic heparinization.

Hepatitis is a complication caused by a virus that is transmitted through blood transfusions and body secretions.

Prevention involves isolation of patients with the virus, strict aseptic technique in access to the patient's bloodstream, careful disposal of needles and blood tubing, attention to environmental cleanliness, and monthly screening of patient and staff for hepatitis virus.

See Appendix B for sample nursing care plan of patients on dialysis.

# CHAPTER 16

# KIDNEY TRANSPLANTATION

The treatment of patients with renal failure has been revolutionized by the recent advances in organ transplantation. The advancement of transplant techniques has raised many pertinent legal, moral, and ethical questions for multidisciplinary study. In this chapter the experience of one patient having a kidney transplant will be described and you will be given an opportunity to consider some features of his nursing care. The routines, methods and treatments differ in each transplant center, so you will gain a general picture, rather than specific knowledge. When you complete this chapter, you should be able to

1. Describe four methods of matching donor and recipient tissues
2. Explain the purpose of immunosuppressive therapy
3. List measures used to preserve a potential cadaveric kidney
4. Explain how and where the donor kidney is grafted to the recipient
5. Recognize signs and symptoms of acute rejection
6. Construct a care plan for the transplant recipient for the first days after surgery.

## Chapter outline

Review of basic information
- The immune response
  - Antigens
  - Antibodies
- Genetic inheritance of tissue types
- Histocompatibility tests
- Rejection of an organ graft

The decision

Preparation for transplant
- X Rays
- Histocompatibility tests
- Surgical preparation

The cadaver donor

Transplantation
- Preoperative care
- The surgical procedure
- Postoperative care
- Episode of acute rejection

# PART I REVIEW

Before studying about kidney transplant, you may wish to review some basic information about the immune system. In transplantation, the donor kidney is an antigen. It stimulates the patient's body to produce antibodies to destroy the graft. Successful transplantation then, depends upon manipulation of this normal defensive system. The nurse needs to understand the basics about immunity in order to plan nursing care for patients whose immune systems are being suppressed.

## Frame 1

The immune response is based on the ability of the white blood cells, especially lymphocytes, to recognize "foreign" substances. The lymphocytes can recognize an invading substance, capture it, and chemically neutralize it.

*Antigen* is a substance (usually protein) that is recognized as foreign and stimulates the immune response. It may be a virus, bacterium, foreign tissue cell, foreign serum, drug, allergen (like pollen), or other substance. Antigens vary in their power to cause the immune response.

*Antibody* is protein formed in the body as the result of white blood cell contact with an antigen. It is also called an immunoglobulin, and it circulates in the blood. It recognizes the antigen and chemically neutralizes it.

Joe Hiller has tuberculosis. Fill in the blanks, completing these statements, which describe the action of the immune response in his case:

1. The antigen is ______________.
2. The white blood cells will produce ______________ to recognize and destroy the bacteria and/or toxins it produces.
3. This immune reaction is helpful to Joe because it ______________.

Answers:

1. tubercule bacillus
2. antibodies
3. destroys the bacteria

## Frame 2

The immune response is an important defense for the body. However, in some cases it impedes treatment. For example, a kidney transplanted into another person are antigenic. Here is a list of some other situations. Choose the ones which could also be antigenic and therefore stimulate an immune response. (If you need a hint, see the list of antigens in Frame 1.)

a. Contact between maternal and fetal blood during separation of the placenta from the uterine wall

b. Immunization for influenza

c. Blood transfusion

d. Antibiotic therapy

e. Liver transplantation

f. All of the above

f

## Frame 3

If a transplanted kidney is to survive, steps must be taken to outwit the patient's immune system. This is done in two main ways

Using donor kidneys that would be the most similar to the patient's.

Using drugs that suppress the immune response (or rejection) in the new kidney.

True or false:

1. ______ The immune system is helpful in long-term survival of transplanted organs.

2. ______ If the donor's tissue protein is similar to the recipient's, it will be a weaker antigen and stimulate less immune response.

1. False

2. True

## Frame 4

The genes present in each cell of the body provide a "blueprint" for the construction of body protein.

Therefore, we would expect that people who have inherited similar genes would have body protein that is structurally similar. The immune response can be "fooled" by a closely matching protein, and may not recognize that it is foreign.

1. Here is a list of possible donors and recipients. Which pair would have the *least* problem with immune response?
   a. Husband-wife
   b. Identical twins
   c. Brother-sister
   d. Cousins
2. How do genes relate to antigens?
   a. Genes are antigens.
   b. Genes destroy antigens.
   c. Genes carry directions for synthesizing proteins which may be antigens.

The genes are arranged on chromosomes as beads are on a string. Each chromosome "string" with its genes from the mother and corresponding genes from the father, are present in each cell of the body.

1. b (They have identical body protein structure.)
2. c

### Frame 5

Research has identified at least 30 antigens in tissues that can trigger rejection of a transplanted kidney. The blueprint area on the gene that relates to the most important of these antigens is called the HLA site (human leukocyte antigen).

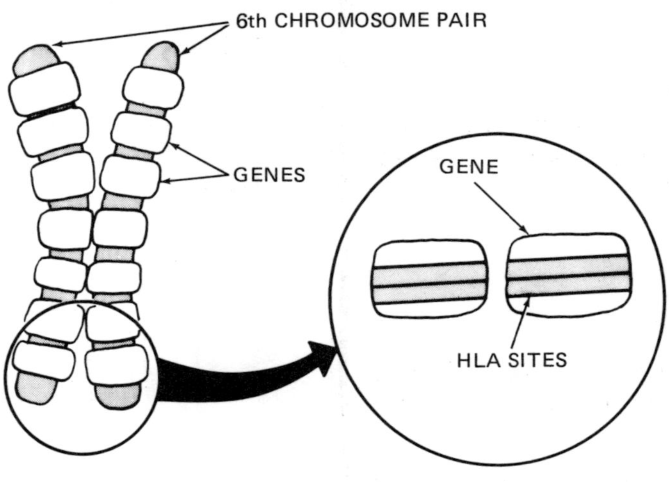


Figure 73

1. How many HLA sites does each person have?

2. Why are the HLA sites important?

1. Four (There are two HLA sites on each strand of the 6th chromosome.)
2. Because they are the blueprint for transplant antigens

**Frame 6**

Each person inherits two HLA sites from each parent. In the diagram below, you can see the possible combinations. (Each letter represents *one* gene with *two HLA sites* on it.)

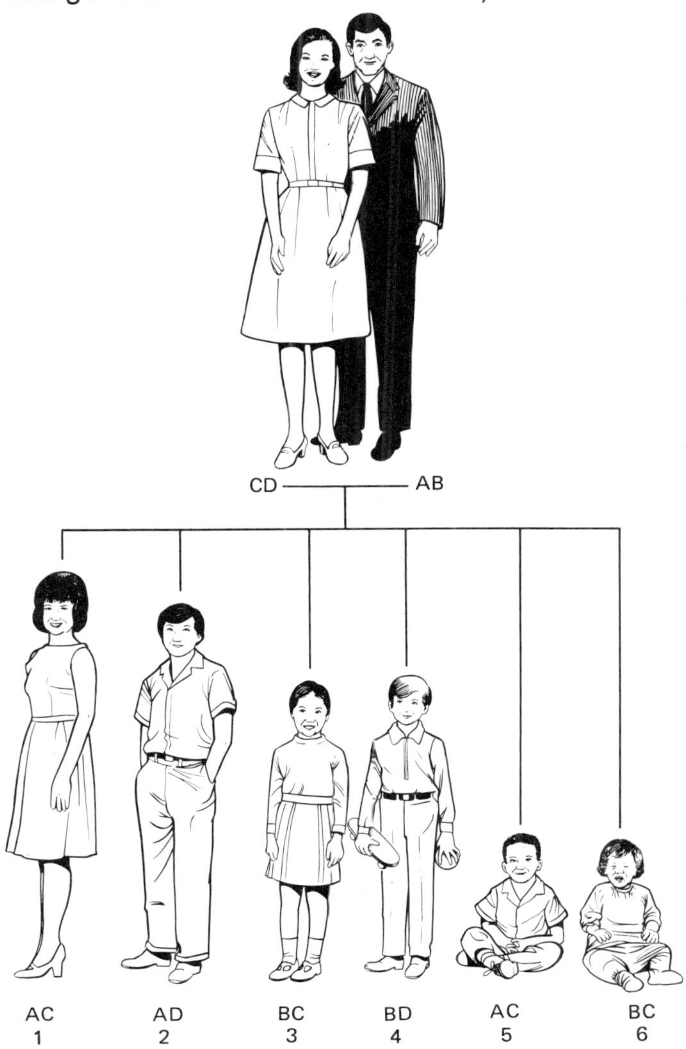


Figure 74

1. Which children have four matching HLA antigens? (Both genes identical)

2. Which people in the family have only 2 matching HLA antigens?
   a. Those with one identical gene
   b. Those with two identical genes

3. Which would offer the best chance for successful transplantation?
   a. Four HLA matches
   b. Two HLA matches
   c. No HLA matches

1. 1 and 5
   3 and 6

2. a (one gene = 2 HLA sites)

3. a

## Frame 7

A series of tests are used to predict the degree of tissue compatibility between donor and recipient. These are called histocompatibility tests.

1. ABO blood typing. Donor and recipient need to be the same blood type. The Rh factor is not relevant.
2. HLA ("tissue") typing. Genes with HLA sites are present in each cell of the body. So the white blood cells (lymphocytes) are used to represent all tissue. The lymphocytes are exposed to a test panel of standardized antigens. If an antigen-antibody response occurs, the cells are destroyed. The response of donor and recipient cells are compared.
3. White cell crossmatch. Recipient serum and donor lymphocytes are mixed. If the recipient has preformed antibodies from past blood transfusions, pregnancies, or infection, these will cause destruction of donor cells. This can also cause graft loss.
4. Mixed leukocyte culture (MLC). White cells from the donor and recipient are cultured together for several days. The immune response is measured by radioactive assay techniques.

1. What are the purposes of histocompatibility tests?
   a. To predict severity of the immune response after transplantation
   b. To show matching of genes that control synthesis of protein
   c. To rule out noncompatible donors
   d. None of the above

1. a, b, c

2. What body cells are used in matching donor and recipient tissue?

2. Red and white blood cells

## Frame 8

Work is constantly in process to improve the sensitivity of histocompatibility tests. However, much is still unknown about the immune response and the specific antigens causing rejection of a grafted kidney.

Now look at how the immune response proceeds after transplantation: circulating lymphocytes pass through the newly implanted kidney, contacting cells whose surfaces bear foreign antigens. The lymphocytes are sensitized and begin to produce antibodies, which destroy the cells of the grafted kidney as they circulate through.

Rejection phenomena are of varying types:

Hyperacute: Tissue destruction occurs within minutes to hours. It is not reversible.

Accelerated: Immune response begins in the first days posttransplantation.

Acute: The immune response causes acute tubular necrosis 2–16 weeks postoperatively.

Chronic: After repeated periods of acute rejection, the graft gradually becomes scarred and loses blood supply. This type ends in removal of the kidney.

True or false:

1. ______ Patients may have some immune response, even if the most compatible donor has been found.

1. True

2. ______ If the rejection episodes are untreated, the cells of the transplanted kidney are destroyed.

2. True

3. ______ Dialysis is never needed after transplantation.

3. False

## Frame 9

The immune response must be suppressed in order to insure survival of the new kidney. The following drugs are commonly used for this purpose:

Azathioprine (Imuran). This drug suppresses the body's response to new tissue antigens. The patient may retain previous immunity to common bacterial and viral infections.

Steroids, especially prednisone. These have antiinflammatory action and may also suppress immune response.

Antilymphocyte globulin (or serum). Human lymphoid tissue is injected into an animal, which produces antibodies against human lymphoid tissue. These antibodies are then given to the patient to suppress his or her lymphoid tissue which causes the immune response to foreign protein.

True or false:

1. ______ Antilymphocyte serum interferes with the body's ability to respond to foreign protein.

1. True

2. ______ The patient on immunosuppressive drugs like azathioprine (Imuran) has no increased risk of infection.

2. False (The patient may acquire infection from new sources. Prednisone also lowers resistance to infection.)

3. ______ The chief action of steroids is to block inflammation and tissue destruction in the graft.

3. True

## Frame 10

Summary:

An antigen is a foreign protein that stimulates an immune response.

An antibody is a protein formed as a result of white blood cell contact with the antigen. It circulates in the blood and chemically neutralizes the antigen. This is called the immune response.

Protein structure is determined by genes. Transplant antigens are related to four human leukocyte antigen (HLA) sites on the 6th chromosome pair.

Transplant donor's and recipient's tissue proteins are matched by ABO blood typing, HLA typing, white cell crossmatch, and mixed leukocyte culture. These tests rule out noncompatible donors by predicting the severity of the immune response.

The immune response causes inflammation with necrosis of the cells of the grafted kidney. Types are

1. Hyperacute—minutes
2. Accelerated—first days
3. Acute—2–16 weeks
4. Chronic—gradual scarring and ischemia

# CASE PRESENTATION PART II THE DECISION

Tim Lewis is a 29-year-old electrician. He has been married to his wife, Donna, for 10 years and has two sons, ages 9 and 7½.

Four years ago, Mr. Lewis found out he had glomerulonephritis and that it was a chronic, progressive problem. For 2 years he was able to control the side effects of chronic renal failure with a medical regimen that included a diet low in protein, sodium, and potassium; fluid restriction that averaged 800 ml/day; and medications to control elevated blood pressure, phosphorus, and potassium.

When this treatment was no longer able to control uremic symptoms, Mr. Lewis began hemodialysis. He had a simple A-V fistula, which was functioning well. He knew that he had three options since he'd reached end-stage renal disease:

> The first option was no further treatment, which would result in certain death. He did not consider this option.
>
> The second option was dialysis for the rest of his life. The physicians discussed this with him, explaining the benefits, possible complications, and quality of life he could expect.
>
> The third option was kidney transplantation. Again the benefits and risks were explained, as well as the statistical probability of a successful transplant.

Tim and Donna Lewis spent long hours discussing dialysis and transplantation. Since he had been on dialysis for a few months, Mr. Lewis was able to judge how this option would work on a long-term basis. He wanted to ski, play tennis, be a Scout leader; now he just didn't have the energy. After working full-time and dialyzing 6 hours, 3 times a week, he was all worn out. He soon made up his mind that he would like a kidney transplant. Six hours, 3 times a week, was a lot of time for a busy man to spend on dialysis, when he could have another choice. And he really didn't like all the venipunctures prior to dialysis.

## Effects of Endstage Renal Disease Treated By Dialysis or Well-Functioning Renal Graft

| EFFECT ON | WITH DIALYSIS | WITH WELL-FUNCTIONING TRANSPLANT |
|---|---|---|
| Renal filtration | Only during dialysis | 24 hours/day |
| Nutrition | Na, K, protein and fluid restrictions | Possible Na restriction for up to 1 year after transplant |
| Erythropoietic system | Anemia, fatigue | Normal red blood cells and hematocrit |
| Skeletal system | Renal osteodystrophy<br>Hyperparathyroidism | No further bone resorption<br>Possible hyperparathyroidism<br>Avascular necrosis |
| Nervous system | Peripheral, gastrointestinal and genitourinary neuropathy | Neuropathy will not progress, and may improve |
| Sexuality | Decreased libido<br>Frequent impotence | Improved libido<br>Impotence may persist |
| Liver | Increased risk of hepatitis from recurrent extracorporeal circulation and transfusion | 10% incidence of hepatitis due to azathioprine therapy |
| Cardiovascular system | Risk of shunt infection, clotting, exsanguination and frequent site changes | No need for vascular access |
| | Accelerated atherosclerosis | Decrease in atherosclerotic Process |
| | Ventricular hypertrophy, heart failure | Ventricular size sometimes returns to normal |
| | Uremic pericarditis | |
| | Cardiac tamponade | |
| Muscular system | Decreased muscle mass due to dietary limits<br>Decreased exercise tolerance | Myopathy which improves when steroid dosage decreases and patient's activity increases |
| Lungs | Risk of pulmonary edema, congestive heart failure | Pulmonary infections secondary to immunosuppressive therapy |
| Dependence | Dependent on machine to support life | Dependent on medications |
| Mortality | 10% for first and second years, 36% for third year and increasing | 20% for first year, then decreases |

From Hudak, Gallo and Lohr, *Critical Care Nursing*, 2nd edition, Philadelphia: J.B. Lippincott, 1977, p. 364

# PART III
# PREPARATION FOR TRANSPLANTATION

A transplant work-up was begun during Mr. Lewis' hospitalization for initiation of dialysis. This included many x rays and special blood tests.

## X rays

These were done to rule out problems that could be aggravated by the immunosuppressive medications Mr. Lewis would need to take when transplanted. If he had cholecystitis, diverticulitis or chronic obstructive lung disease, the use of immunosuppressives could result in fulminating infection. Long-term steroid therapy carries the risk of gastrointestinal bleeding, so x rays were done to rule out ulcers and gastritis. Mr. Lewis' lower urinary tract (ureters, bladder, and urethra) were x rayed for any structural anomalies that would affect the transplantation.

## Histocompatibility Tests

Mr. Lewis' blood was subjected to the following tests:

Red blood cell type—A
HLA antigens

His family was also evaluated for potential donors. In this transplant center, all family members were tested. Then each person was interviewed by a member of the team and asked whether he or she was willing to donate a kidney. Those unwilling to donate were not included in the list of matching donors. Here are the results of the tests:

Mother—Blood type B
Father—Blood type A, 5-year history of hypertension
Brother—Blood type A, 3 HLA antigen match
Sister—Blood type AB
Sister—Blood type A, 2 HLA antigen match } unwilling
Sister—Blood type A, 4 HLA antigen match } to donate

Mr. Lewis' father's history of hypertension ruled him out as a donor. The mother and the sister with AB blood are not suitable donors since their B antigens would react with Mr. Lewis' A type blood. Since the other two sisters were unwilling to donate, Mr. Lewis' brother was the only person to be further evaluated as a donor.

The potential living related donor is thoroughly evaluated to document that he has two normally functioning kidneys and is free of underlying disease.

*Panel 1*

*Criteria for Selection of Living Donors*

1. *Voluntary donation without coercion.*
2. *Stable social and psychological history.*
3. *Complete history and physical examination normal.*
4. *Absence of renal disease, hypertension, significant diabetes, or transmittable neoplasm.*
5. *Normal CBC, ECG, chest x ray, SMA-12, coagulation profile, STS.*
6. *Normal intravenous urogram.*
7. *Normal creatinine clearance.*
8. *Negative urine culture on two occasions; normal urinalysis.*
9. *Normal aortogram and renal arteriograms (major renal anomalies or more than two renal arteries may exclude donor).*
10. *Compatible ABO typing.*
11. *Compatible HLA tissue typing.*
12. *Negative cross-match with recipient.*

*Colberg, JE. "Selection and Management of Patients for Renal Transplantation," Surgical Clinics of North America* 53: *685, 1973.*

Mr. Lewis' brother had an extensive work-up including blood tests for hematocrit and creatinine, and a creatinine clearance, which were all normal. The chest x ray was negative, but the renal arteriogram showed a narrowing of the left renal artery. This eliminated Mr. Lewis' brother as a potential donor.

The elimination of all willing potential family donors was depressing to the whole family. Mr. Lewis' name was added to the growing list of dialysis patients waiting for a cadaver transplant. The physician explained that there is a nationwide registry of patients waiting for organs donated at the time of death. The patient with the best HLA match gets the available kidney.

## Surgical Preparation

Splenectomy and nephrectomy are two surgical procedures that may need to be performed prior to the transplantation. Splenectomy is done to help "turn off" the body's natural immune mechanisms.

Nephrectomy is done if the kidneys are infected (polycystic kidneys or pyelonephritis) or if they're contributing to uncontrolled hypertension.

Mr. Lewis required splenectomy but not nephrectomy.

# PART IV
# THE CADAVER DONOR

In each transplant center, there is a continuous list of people who are waiting for a kidney from a cadaver donor. The need for these organs is far above the number provided. The use of cadaver donors allows living related donors to be well-matched.

In a small city, 150 miles from Mr. Lewis' home, 19-year-old Nancy Holmes was in a motorcycle accident. She received a severe blow to her head and was comatose with Cheyne–Stokes respirations when admitted to the local emergency room. She was placed on a respirator and transferred to ICU.

During the next 24 hours, Ms. Holmes' neurologic status steadily declined, until she had no spontaneous movement, no spontaneous respiration, and no brainstem reflexes such as pupil changes, corneal reflex, gag reflex, or tonic neck reflexes. The next day, the physician talked to Ms. Holmes' parents about the hopelessness of the situation.

Joanne Windham was assigned as the primary nurse in ICU. In order to help the family to understand the neurologic concept of brain death, she

Allowed the family to observe her assess the patient's neurologic reactions

Let them be there when the respirator was removed for 4-minute test periods

Allowed them time to ventilate their feelings and ask questions.

Later in the day, Mrs. Holmes said, "If only some good could come out of this situation! Our daughter was so active, so full of life. She once said if she died that it would be nice if someone could use her kidneys. Could you find out if this would be possible?"

Joanne contacted the family's physician. Together they initiated a plan to save the kidneys. the physician contacted the Transplant Center with information about the donor's present condition, age, blood type, and renal function. (Potential donors should be under age 55–65 and should be free of infection and cancer. They should not have a history of renal disease, hypertension or a systemic disease such as diabetes mellitus.)

Ms. Holmes' irreversible brain damage was further confirmed by two flat electroencephalograms, done at 24-hour intervals. She was pronounced dead, and her family signed the consent authorizing organ donation.

Joanne's role included supporting Mr. and Mrs. Holmes through this crisis and maintaining the donor kidneys in optimal condition.

Cell perfusion in the kidneys was supported by

1. Maintaining the blood pressure at an effective level through the use of IV fluids, and vasopressors if necessary
2. Oxygenation of the blood by means of the respirator

Urine output was maintained at approximately 100 ml/hour through the use of fluids, plasma expanders, and diuretics.

The organ procurement team arrived from the transplantation center. The donor body was given a rapid infusion of normal saline containing sodium bicarbonate and heparin to expand fluid volume and prevent acidosis. Vasoconstriction of the renal vessels was prevented by giving an alpha-adrenergic blocker 30 minutes before discontinuing the respirator.

The donor nephrectomy was done in an operating room. The family physician disconnected the respirator and the donor nephrectomy began 5 minutes after the cardiac arrest and was completed within 60 minutes. Both kidneys and ureters were removed with a segment of aorta and vena cava.

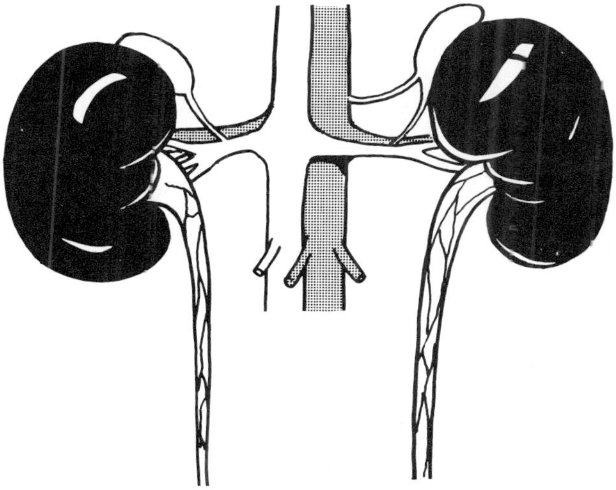

Figure 75

The excised kidneys were preserved for use by the following procedure:

1. Immediately after nephrectomy, the kidneys were placed in a basin of cold sterile saline in which multiple sterile iced saline cubes were placed to maintain temperature.
2. The renal arteries were then cannulated and the kidneys flushed with 4°C medicated Ringer's lactate containing sodium bicarbonate, penicillin, heparin, and steroids.
3. When clear effluent was flushed from the renal vein, lactate flush was discontinued and the kidneys were placed in the preservation apparatus and brought to the transplantation hospital by the organ procurement team.

# PART V TRANSPLANTATION

## Preoperative Care

Mr. Lewis was at work when he received a call that a kidney with a suitable tissue match was available. After months of dreaming about this call, and after one cancellation because of the presence of preformed antigens, it now seemed somehow unreal. It was an exciting drive to the hospital. He thought, "Would it really match this time? If I only can get off dialysis! What if the kidney rejects me!"

Mr. Lewis was admitted directly to the dialysis unit for a dialysis run before surgery. Blood studies checked included CBC, creatinine, urea nitrogen, electrolytes, Prothrombin time, hepatitis B surface antigen (Australian antigen), blood typing and crossmatch for 3 units fresh frozen washed cells, and a final crossmatch for circulating antibodies. A positive test for antibodies could cancel the transplant procedure. (A recent viral infection is an example of a situation that could create new circulating antibodies.)

Mr. Lewis' hemoglobin was 7.1 mg/100 ml. The 3 units of fresh frozen washed cells would give him an extra supply of RBCs that would help him until his transplanted kidney would be able to stimulate RBC production—about 3 months.

Preoperatively, Mr. Lewis was also begun on immunosuppressive medications. He was given azothioprine (Imuran) 2–3 mg/kg and prednisone 1.5–2.0 mg/kg. The antacid he had been taking with meals to bind phosphorus was discontinued and he was begun on magaldrate (Riopan) 30 ml between meals and at bedtime to protect the gastric mucosa.

Anne, Mr. Lewis' dialysis nurse, was trying to review with him what would happen once he was through with his dialysis treatment. He found it hard to concentrate because his mind kept wandering to "Won't it be wonderful if . . .," but he tried to listen as he knew his cooperation would help make this transplantation a success.

Anne told Mr. Lewis all about his preop preparation:

> We're starting you on nothing by mouth now. As soon as you've completed dialyzing, you'll go to your room. There you will receive an enema of plain water to cleanse the lower bowel of stool. You will shower using a special soap that slows the growth of bacteria. As soon as you're ready, you will receive two medications by injection to prepare you for anesthesia. One shot will make you sleepy and the other will dry the secretions in your mouth and throat.
>
> In the operating room they'll shave your front from the nipples to your knees. You'll also have a catheter inserted into your bladder. This will help insure that your urine can be freely passed after surgery. We can monitor the amount more frequently and it helps determine how much fluid you'll need replaced by IVs. Frequently, as the kidneys begin to work you may put out large amounts of water. The catheter will be left in place for about a week.

Anne also reviewed with Mr. Lewis the placement of the kidney. She helped Mr. Lewis practice the techniques of deep breathing and coughing. He realized their importance because he'd had pneumonia when his splenectomy was done. Tim knew that as soon as he was able, he'd begin to get food and fluids by mouth. He also knew that special mouth care was important in preventing infection, especially while he was on the high dosages of immunosuppressive medications. They also discussed the probable need for dialysis after surgery to help correct homeostasis until the new kidney was functioning.

Mr. Lewis' wife, Donna, was included in this teaching situation. Anne also offered her support when she found her crying in the waiting room.

## The Surgical Procedure

After induction of anesthesia, Mr. Lewis' skin preparation was completed and an indwelling catheter was inserted. The catheter protects the bladder suture lines by allowing continuous urine drainage.

An oblique incision was made extending from the 11th rib to several centimeters above the symphysis pubis. The peritoneum was not opened. To implant the kidney, the surgeon anastomosed the donor renal artery to Mr. Lewis' external iliac artery. The donor renal vein was connected to his external iliac vein. The new kidney lies in the iliac fossa.

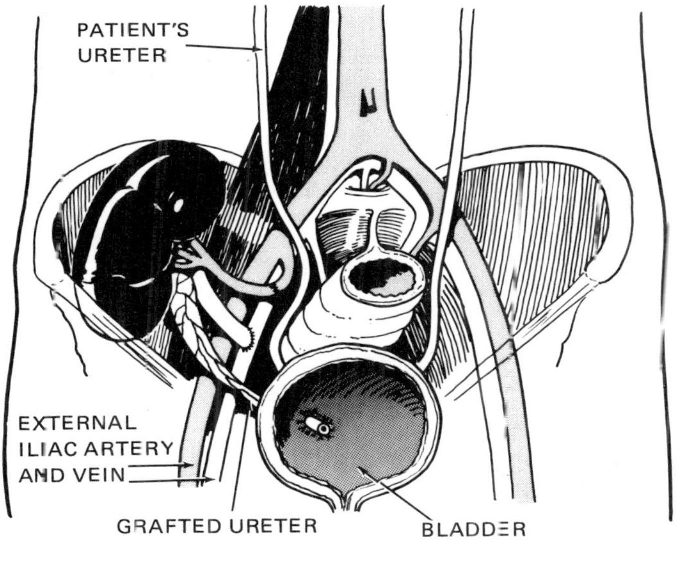


Figure 76

The donor ureter was then implanted into the posterior wall of Mr. Lewis' bladder through a submucosal tunnel. This tunnel acts as a valve and prevents reflex of urine into the kidney.

The surgeon then removed the blood vessel clamps and Mr. Lewis' new kidney became pink and firm. Within a few minutes the kidney began making urine.

## Postop Care

Ellen admitted Mr. Lewis to the renal ICU. She noted that he was easily aroused, and he did not complain of pain. She checked the IV lines, noting type of solution, flow rate and venipuncture site. His catheter had drained 900 ml since revascularization of the graft. His vital signs were stable and within normal limits and his fistula was patent. There was no drainage on his dressing.

After getting Mr. Lewis settled and arranging for his wife to see him, Ellen reviewed the chart to note the preop lab reports, the surgical report, and orders for IVs and medications. She began a nursing care plan that featured the following goals:

1. Maintain fluid and electrolyte balance.
2. Maintain adequate level of urine output.
3. Prevent infection.
4. Recognize signs of rejection.
5. Provide information on procedures and feedback about clinical condition to the patient and his wife.
6. Prevent clotting of fistula.

## Discussion

Now think about choosing nursing interventions to meet the goals of Mr. Lewis' care.

*Problem 1*

Use the Response Indicator below to choose the nursing actions that are directed toward maintaining adequate urine output and drainage. Squares numbered: ____________

*Problem 2*

Which nursing actions focus on maintaining the balance of fluid and electrolytes? Squares numbered: ____________

*Problem 3*

Infection is a grave concern in the transplant patient. Choose the interventions that are aimed at diminishing the risk of infection postop. Squares numbered: ____________

| Response Indicator | | | | |
|---|---|---|---|---|
| IV—replace urine output ml for ml hourly plus 30 ml for insensible loss to a maximum 200 ml/hour 1 | Restrict visiting No persons with colds or infection 2 | Note any decrease in urine output or a change in color 3 | Begin ambulation first postop day 4 | Weigh patient each morning 5 |
| Mouth care p.c. and h.s. with antifungal swish-and-swallow routine 6 | Note intake and output 7 | Sterile bladder irrigation with normal saline p.r.n. if output decreases 8 | Medicate for pain 9 | Advance diet as tolerated (no longer protein or potassium restricted) 10 |
| Patient to wear gown and mask if leaving the patient care area 11 | Milk the urinary catheter 12 | Check blood and urine test results, K and Na, report abnormalities 13 | Turn, cough, hyperventilate every 1-2 hours, blow bottles, postural drainage if needed 14 | Check dressings for drainage every 2-4 hours (mark boundaries, change if wet) 15 |
| Check the catheter for kinks 16 | Special catheter and perineal care every 8 hours 17 | Breath sounds every 4 hours 18 | Vital signs every 2-4 hours (blood pressure, pulse, central venous pressure) 19 | |

## Comments

*Problem 1* — Urinary Output

Suggested responses: 1, 3, 4, 7, 8, 12, 14, 15, 16

O 1, 3, 7

Careful assessment of input and output patterns can pick up possible complications. A decreased urine output, especially after a period of diuresis, could be from a kink in the drainage tubing or from a clot. Dehydration or hypovolemia are systemic causes of a decreased output, and the new kidney is a prime candidate for acute tubular necrosis. Keeping

| Response Indicator | | | | |
|---|---|---|---|---|
| IV—replace urine output ml for ml hourly plus 30 ml for insensible loss to a maximum 200 ml/hour 1 | Restrict visiting No persons with colds or infection 2 | Note any decrease in urine output or a change in color 3 | Begin ambulation first postop day 4 | Weigh patient each morning 5 |
| Mouth care p.c. and h.s. with antifungal swish-and-swallow routine 6 | Note intake and output 7 | Sterile bladder irrigation with normal saline p.r.n. if output decreases 8 | Medicate for pain 9 | Advance diet as tolerated (no longer protein or potassium restricted) 10 |
| Patient to wear gown and mask if leaving the patient care area 11 | Milk the urinary catheter 12 | Check blood and urine test results, K and Na, report abnormalities 13 | Turn, cough, hyperventilate every 1-2 hours, blow bottles, postural drainage if needed 14 | Check dressings for drainage every 2-4 hours (mark boundaries, change if wet) 15 |
| Check the catheter for kinks 16 | Special catheter and perineal care every 8 hours 17 | Breath sounds every 4 hours 18 | Vital signs every 2-4 hours (blood pressure, pulse, central venous pressure) 19 | |

IV replacement therapy on time is important in providing for an adequate output. Decreased urine output could also be from a ureteral obstruction or from a renal artery or vein thrombosis.

O 8, 12, 16

Decreased urine output could be due to problems with the drainage tubing. Check for kinks, then try milking the tubing and, if ordered, irrigate with sterile normal saline (an antibiotic may also be used in the solution).

O 15

Urine may be draining from the ureteral anastomosis site rather than the catheter. Evidence of this would be urine drainage on the dressings. This leakage, especially in the presence of a decreased urine output, could indicate urine retention, perhaps from a problem mentioned in the first comment. Technical and surgical complications have been reported as causing a 10% loss of graft function.

O 4, 14

Activity should also encourage proper drainage.

*Problem 2* — Fluid and Electrolyte Balance

Suggested responses: 1, 5, 7, 10, 13, 19

O 1, 5, 7, 19

Each transplant situation is unique as the kidney's output cannot be predicted. For some there is initial diuresis, for others, oliguria or anuria. Intravenous intake is provided until the patient can take fluids by mouth. Weight, vital signs, and intake and output patterns all help assess the state of fluid balance.

O 10, 13

A potassium imbalance is the most commonly seen electrolyte problem posttransplantation. If the kidney graft is functioning and excreting a large urine volume, it can usually excrete the excessive potassium caused by tissue damage during the surgery. In oliguria or anuria situa-

| Response Indicator | | | | |
|---|---|---|---|---|
| IV—replace urine output ml for ml hourly plus 30 ml for insensible loss to a maximum 200 ml/hour 1 | Restrict visiting No persons with colds or infection 2 | Note any decrease in urine output or a change in color 3 | Begin ambulation first postop day 4 | Weigh patient each morning 5 |
| Mouth care p.c. and h.s. with antifungal swish-and-swallow routine 6 | Note intake and output 7 | Sterile bladder irrigation with normal saline p.r.n. if output decreases 8 | Medicate for pain 9 | Advance diet as tolerated (no longer protein or potassium restricted) 10 |
| Patient to wear gown and mask if leaving the patient care area 11 | Milk the urinary catheter 12 | Check blood and urine test results, K and Na, report abnormalities 13 | Turn, cough, hyperventilate every 1–2 hours, blow bottles, postural drainage if needed 14 | Check dressings for drainage every 2–4 hours (mark boundaries, change if wet) 15 |
| Check the catheter for kinks 16 | Special catheter and perineal care every 8 hours 17 | Breath sounds every 4 hours 18 | Vital signs every 2–4 hours (blood pressure, pulse, central venous pressure) 19 | |

tions, Kayexalate or dialysis may be used to decrease serum potassium. The potassium may also need to be controlled in the diet.

I 3, 15

You may have also included noting a decrease in urine output as relevant to fluid and electrolyte balance and your reasoning is probably correct. If dressings have heavy amounts of fluid drainage, it would be wise to weigh them and include this output in the replacement calculations.

*Problem 3* — Prevention of Infection

Suggested responses: 2, 3, 4, 6, 11, 14, 15, 17, 18

O 2, 4, 11, 14, 18

Transplant patients are susceptible to any kind of infection. Exposure to others with upper respiratory infection, for example, should be avoided. Early postop activities to promote good ventilation and pulmonary hygiene are important. Use assessment of breath sounds to determine efficiency of the pulmonary hygiene program.

O 3, 6, 15, 17

The immunosuppressive drugs necessary for graft survival make even normal organisms become a foe. The bladder and perineal care is probably the area of most concern. The catheter usually remains in the bladder 7 days to avoid any pressure on the anastomosis site. A bacteriostatic and/or antiseptic cleansing of the perineum and the catheter should be done every 8–12 hours.

Wet dressings are an excellent media for growing microorganisms. Use of antibiotics and immunosuppressives can alter the normal flora of the mouth and cause infection.

I 8, 9, 10

You may have included these three interventions. You were correct if your reasoning included *1*) emphasis on the sterility of the bladder irrigation, *2*) the fact that a pain-free patient could cooperate more fully with turning, coughing, and walking and *3*) a good diet should promote healing and strengthen the patient against bacterial invasion.

# CASE PRESENTATION

## Episode of Acute Rejection

By the third postop day, Mr. Lewis' temperature was 101°F. His blood pressure had risen from 130/70 to 148/90. His serum creatinine was now 2.1 mg/100 ml when it had been 1.8 mg/100 ml two days postop. His urine output decreased from 900 to 500 ml/day.

Ellen was concerned about these symptoms, because they are common during episodes of rejection.

### Signs and Symptoms of Rejection

*Physical*

1. Decrease in urine output
2. Weight gain
3. Increased blood pressure
4. Generalized edema
5. Temperature of 100°F and higher
6. General malaise
7. Tenderness over the graft site
8. Swelling of the graft

*Laboratory Values*

9. Increased serum creatinine
10. Decreased urine creatinine and creatinine clearance
11. Proteinuria
12. Increased BUN
13. Increased serum sodium

## Frame 11

From the list of common signs and symptoms of rejection, check the ones that Mr. Lewis had. 1, 3, 5, 9

His symptoms could *also* be caused by which of these problems? a, b, c

a. Acute tubular necrosis
b. Fluid overload
c. Infection
d. None of the above

In order to plan further care, the physicians ordered a renal scan. Mr. Lewis went to the nuclear medicine department, where a radioactive isotope was injected into a vein. The technician took photographs for the next ½ hour to show renal uptake and excretion of the isotope. A normal kidney rapidly filters the isotope and excretes it. During acute rejection, uptake is slow and irregular, and excretion of the isotope decreases. During acute tubular necrosis there is isotope uptake, but no excretion.

Mr. Lewis' renogram showed decreased rate of isotope uptake, slower transit through the nephrons, and decreased excretion of the isotope into the collection system.

The physicians then began to treat Mr. Lewis for acute rejection. At this time he was on the following immunosuppressive medication schedule:

1. Solu-Medrol—IV drip

   | | |
   |---|---|
   | Day 1: 1 g | Day 5: 250 mg |
   | Day 2: 1 g | Day 6: 250 mg |
   | Day 3: 500 mg | Day 7: 125 mg |
   | Day 4: 500 mg | Day 8: 125 mg |

2. After the Solu-Medrol was discontinued, prednisone would be given, beginning with 60 mg daily and then in decreasing dosages until 15 mg was reached and used for maintenance.
3. Azothioprine (Imuran) 150 mg daily (2.5 mg/kg)

Mr. Lewis received the scheduled dose of Solu-Medrol 500 mg in the morning.

In the afternoon he received an extra 0.5 g. The Solu-Medrol course was then restarted at the beginning. He received a dose of Kayexalate because his serum potassium was 5.8 mEq/liter.

The next day, his urine output was under 500 ml/day (average 20 ml/hour), his creatinine was 2.4 mg/100 ml, and his potassium was back to 5.9 mEq/liter. The physicians decided that Mr. Lewis needed to be dialyzed. Even though he had known this was a possibility, it was very difficult for him to face dialysis again. "What if I'll need to continue?" he'd asked Ellen.

## Frame 12

What can Ellen do to support Mr. Lewis during this time of dialysis?

a. Explain what rejection is and what steps are being taken to combat it.
b. Allow him time to ventilate his feelings.
c. Assure him that the need to dialyze is temporary.
d. Recognize that depression is a normal reaction.

a, b, d (If the rejection episode cannot be reversed, Mr. Lewis will be on chronic dialysis again.)

Mr. Lewis was dialyzed twice during the next week. During this time of rejection, the physicians also irradiated his kidney on three alternate days. This treatment decreases the number of lymphocytes attacking the graft.

The favorable response to treatment was soon manifested by a decrease in blood pressure. His urine output increased and his lab values returned to normal.

If Mr. Lewis' kidney had not responded to the antirejection therapy, the doctors would have to assess if this was acute or chronic rejection. Chronic rejection is conservatively managed without increasing immunosuppression, and the patient ultimately returns to hemodialysis. (The kidney graft is left in place unless the patient would develop hypertension or an infection. He would then be considered a candidate for retransplantation.)

Important self-care routines were reviewed with Mr. Lewis while he was hospitalized: how and when to check his blood pressure, pulse, temperature, weight, and height. Medication schedules were established as well as guidelines for him to use in deciding when to contact the transplantation clinic.

Twelve days after receiving his kidney, Mr. Lewis left the hospital. He knew that the next days, weeks, and months meant close contact with the transplantation team for monitoring and preventing complications. But Mr. Lewis definitely felt it was worth it. He felt stronger, he didn't have to be tied to the dialyzer for 18 hours a week, and his only diet restriction was low sodium to help prevent steroid-induced edema.

Mr. Lewis is aware that his appearance may change from the medications. He may gain weight and his face may be moonlike. He also knows that his emotions may become unpredictable due to an effect of the medications. He's living with the knowledge that someday his kidney may be rejected, but he is not letting that interfere with his plans. He's set out to work, play, and enjoy his family in the fullest way possible.

## Frame 13

Summary:

Kidney transplantation is frequently chosen as the method to replace loss of normal kidney function. It is favored over dialysis in that a more normal life-style, with fewer medical complications, can be resumed.

Sources of kidneys are: *1*) living related donors (sibling, parent, child) who have normally functioning kidneys and no underlying disease; *2*) cadaver donors who are free of infection and cancer and do not have a history of renal disease or hypertension.

The donor and recipient tissue proteins are matched for ABO blood type, HLA antigens, white cell crossmatch and a mixed leukocyte culture.

The transplant recipient may have had a splenectomy to help decrease the body's natural defense mechanism and a nephrectomy if the kidneys are infected or contributing to hypertension.

The transplant kidney is placed in the iliac fossa which brings it to close proximity with the urinary bladder.

Postop nursing goals:

1. Maintain fluid and electrolyte balance.
2. Maintain adequate levels of urine output.
3. Prevent infection.
4. Recognize signs of infection.

Graft survival is maintained with daily immunosuppressive drug therapy. Two common medications are azathioprine (Imuran) and prednisone.

Two common complications are rejection and infection. Ongoing nursing care involves detection and prevention of these problems. See Appendix B for sample care plan.

# APPENDIX A
## Admission Assessment Form — End-Stage Renal Failure

Name ______________________ Admission Date ______________________

Age ________ Sex ________ Religion ______________________

Marital Status ______________________ Children (ages) ______________________

______________________

Height ______________________ T ________ P ________ R ________

Weight: Present ______________________ BP: Supine ________ AP: Supine ________

Usual ______________________ Standing ________ Standing ________

---

1. Renal—Urinary Output
   a. Color ______________________
   b. Amount ______________________
   c. ____Nocturia ____Burning
      ____Frequency ____Distention
      ____Urgency ____Retention
      ____Pain ____Foamy

2. Cardiac
   a. See BPs above
   b. Irregular pulse ________
   c. Pericardial friction rub ________
   d. Other abnormal heart sounds ________
   e. Chest pain ________
   f. Pulsus paradoxus ________
   g. Other: ______________________

3. Body Fluids
   a. See weights above
   b. Edema:
      ____Slight ____Feet ____Sacrum
      ____Moderate ____Ankles ____Abdomen
      ____Pitting ____Legs ____Periorbital

4. Respiratory
   a. Rate ________ b. Depth ________
   c. Odor ______________________
   d. Breathing difficulties
      Dyspnea: ____Bedrest ____Walking
      ____Sitting ____Stairs
      ____Cheyne Stokes ____Kussmaul
      ____Other: ______________________
   e. Cough: ____Moist
      ____Hacking
      ____Productive
   f. Lung sounds: ____Clear ____Rales
      ____Moist ____Wheezes

5. Neural
   a. Mental status: ____Alert ____Confused
      ____Drowsy ____Comatose
      ____Inattentive ____Forgetful
      ____Other: ______________________
   b. Orientation to time, place, person ________

5. (Continued)
   c. Sensory disturbances: ____Visual ____Olfactory
      ____Auditory ____Tactile
   d. Motor disturbances:
      Gait (difficulty walking) ______________________
      Tingling ______________________
   e. Other ______________________

6. Gastrointestinal
   a. Mouth ____Dry ____Ulcers
   b. Appetite: ______________________
      ____Anorexia ____Nausea ____Vomiting
      Best meal ______________________
   c. ____Indigestion ____Diarrhea
      ____Pain ____Constipation
      ____Hiccups ____Blood in stool
      ____Coffee-ground emesis

7. Skin
   a. Color ______________________
      ____Pallor ____Jaundice
      ____Cyanotic ____Gray brown
      ____Pruritus ____Bruises
      ____Lesions ____Crystals
      ____Dryness
   b. Perspiration:
      Increased____ Normal____ Decreased____

8. Musculoskeletal
   a. Muscles: ____Good tone ____Flaccid
      ____Atrophy ____"Renal flap"
      ____Cramps
      Other: ______________________
   b. Skeletal: ____Pain ____Fractures

9. Endocrine
   ____Delayed puberty ____Decreased potency
   ____Decreased libido
   ____Amenorrhea

10. Behavior on admission
    ____Apprehensive/anxious ____Discouraged
    ____Restless/agitated ____Withdrawn
    ____Irritable ____Depressed
    ____Demanding ____Calm
    ____Other: ______________________

# APPENDIX B
# General Nursing Care Plan

## END-STAGE RENAL FAILURE

| Problem | Desired Outcome | Nursing Action/Order |
|---|---|---|
| I. Maintenance of fluid balance<br><br>Avoid<br><br>Hypervolemia and hypovolemia<br>Pulmonary edema<br>Congestive heart failure | A. Fluid intake is adjusted as indicated by patient's condition (i.e., every hour, every 2 hours, every 4 hours) to meet the patient's requirements<br><br>B. Imbalances detected early | 1. Daily weight—same time, same scale, same clothes<br>2. Accurate I and O—minimum every 8 hours to include<br>Intake—IV's, oral, gastric feedings<br>Output—urine, nasogastric suction, stool, drainage, emesis, diaphoresis<br>3. Assess edema—minimum every 8 hours: pedal, sacral, periorbital; check skin turgor<br>4. Administer diuretics as ordered; observe for response to diuretic (know action and time of action)<br>5. BP, P, CVP, PCWP (Swan-Ganz) monitor every 4 hours minimum; PAP every hour (Swan-Ganz catheter)<br>6. Check heart and lung sounds minimum every 8 hours; check for distention of jugular neck veins |
| II. Maintenance of electrolyte balance<br><br>Avoid<br><br>Hyperkalemia and hypokalemia<br>Hypernatremia and hyponatremia<br>Hypocalcemia<br>Hyperphosphatemia | A. Electrolytes exchanged by the kidney remain within normal limits:<br>K+ 3.5–5.5 mEq/liter<br>Na+ 135–145 mEq/liter<br>Cl- 98–102 mEq/liter<br>Mg++ 1.5–2.5 mEq/liter<br>$PO_4$ 2.45-4.5 mg/100 ml<br>Ca++ 8–10 mg/100 ml<br><br>B. Imbalances detected early<br><br>C. Avoid losses of fluid that contain electrolytes | 1. Collect laboratory specimens accurately<br>2. Be aware of electrolyte concentration of IV's and medications<br>3. Observe for signs of<br>Dysrhythmias—ECG monitor changes<br>Hyponatremia—weakness<br>Hypernatremia—increased thirst<br>Hypocalcemia—tetany<br>positive Chvostek's sign<br>4. Hyperkalemia—administer Kayexalate *oral*—can be mixed with sorbitol for osmotic diuresis by pharmacy; *enema*—retained for 30 to 45 minutes<br>5. Hyperphosphatemia—administer phosphate-binder with meals for full utilization of binding effect; do not give iron and mineral supplements with the phosphate-binder as it will bind them too.<br>6. Reinforce diet low in Na+ and N+ |

## END-STAGE RENAL FAILURE, CONTINUED

| Problem | Desired Outcome | Nursing Action/Order |
|---|---|---|
| III. Maintenance of acid–base balance | A. Bicarbonate ($HCO_3$), pH of blood and urine, $CO_2$ content, remain in normal range:<br>$HCO_3$ 21–29 mEq/liter<br>pH 7.35–7.45<br>$CO_2$ content 22–30 mEq/liter<br>urine pH avg 6.0 (4.6–8.0 depending on diet)<br>B. Imbalances detected early | 1. Observe for increased rate and depth of respiration; decrease in mental alertness (confusion, lethargy, coma)<br>2. Administer bicarbonate or precursors of bicarbonate as ordered |
| IV. Coping with side effects of abnormal solute excretion—evidenced by an increased serum urea and creatinine clearance | A. Early detection of azotemia | 1. Record amount and color of urine<br>2. Assess for nocturia, frequency, urgency, pain, burning, distention, retention, foamy urine<br>3. Note and report abnormal urine specific gravity and osmolality, hematuria, proteinuria, increased BUN, increased creatinine, increased uric acid, decreased creatinine clearance<br>4. See Problems VI through XIII for specific problems and actions |
| V. Promotion of protein homeostasis | A. Prevent a state of negative nitrogen balance (catabolism) | 1. Encourage diet as ordered:<br>*Low protein* to decrease urea, uric acid blood levels<br>*High in calories* to spare protein<br>Plan meal with patient<br>Six small feedings<br>2. Proper administration of total parenteral nutrition if ordered |

## END-STAGE RENAL FAILURE, CONTINUED

| Problem | Desired Outcome | Nursing Action/Order |
|---|---|---|
| VI. Cardiac problems<br><br>CHF<br>Arrhythmias (hyporkalemia)<br>Pericarditis<br>Circulatory collapse | A. Prevention of cardiac problems | 1. CHF—assess for and report<br>Increase in blood pressure, weight, tissue edema, jugular vein distention, CVP<br>Unusual cardiac rhythms (gallop, tachycardia)<br>2. Dysrhythmias (increased K)—assess for and report<br>Spiked T waves<br>Wide QRS interval<br>Also symptoms of CHF (#1)<br>Have available:<br>a. Ion exchange resins (Kayexalate) for oral or retention enema; use to decrease K+ in the bowel<br>b. Hypertonic glucose solutions and regular insulin to move K+ back into the cells<br>c. Sodium bicarbonate to correct acidosis and 10% calcium gluconate to modify cardiac irritability<br>3. Pericarditis—assess for and report:<br>Low grade fever (less than 100°F)<br>Paradoxic pulse greater than normal (6–10)<br>Pericardial friction rub<br>Distant heart sounds<br>Chest pain, worse if lying flat, relieved if sitting upright, and leaning forward<br>Have equipment available for a pericardiocentesis<br>4. Circulatory collapse—assess for sudden decrease in BP and CVP; weak, thready pulse; tachycardia; diaphoresis; cold extremities; decreased mental alertness |
| VII. Respiratory problems<br>Pulmonary edema<br>Pneumonia | A. Prevention of respiratory problems | 1. Assess for changes in rate, depth, and regularity of respirations, e.g., dyspnea, orthopnea<br>2. Note changes in lung sounds, i.e., wet rales<br>3. Report cyanosis, severe restlessness, blood-tinged or frothy mucus.<br>4. If confined to bed, turn, cough, deep breathe every 2–4 hours; blow bottles every 4 hours<br>5. Promote early ambulation<br>6. Monitor arterial blood gases and chest x rays |

## END-STAGE RENAL FAILURE, CONTINUED

| Problem | Desired Outcome | Nursing Action/Order |
|---|---|---|
| VIII. Neural problems<br>Decreased mentation<br><br>Sensory disturbances<br>Motor disturbances | A. Reduce patient's anxiety due to changes in mental status<br><br>B. Protect from injury<br><br>C. Maintain current level of mobility | 1. Check orientation to time, place, person, minimum every 8 hours<br>2. Check for mentation changes, i.e., alert, drowsy, inattentive, confused, forgetful, inability to concentrate<br>3. Talk with patient for short periods of time<br>4. Give only small amounts of information at a time<br>5. Have patience for need to frequently repeat and review information and instructions<br>6. Assure patient and family that this should improve after dialysis is started<br>7. Evaluate patient's vision, hearing, smell, touch<br>8. Assess for motor problems:<br>Difficulty walking (gait)<br>Tingling or numbness in walking<br>9. Provide a safe environment<br>10. Assist with personal care and activity as patient's disability indicates |
| IX. Gastrointestinal problems<br><br>Mouth — bad "metallic" taste, dryness, potential ulcerations | A. Decrease of discomfort due to symptoms | 1. Assist patient with mouth care a.c., p.c., and h.s. (prn)<br>Use mouthwashes<br>2. Offer hard candies, gum<br>3. Use ice chips instead of water<br>4. Viscous Xylocaine mouthwash for painful oral lesions<br>5. Substitute gauze for toothbrush if bleeding from gums |
| Nausea and vomiting | B. Prevention of nausea and vomiting<br>Patient eats foods offered<br><br>C. Documented increase in food intake | 6. Administer antiemetics 30 — 45 min before meals<br>7. Use antacids if they help patient<br>8. Dietician consult<br>a. Small frequent feedings<br>b. Foods patient can chew and swallow<br>c. Supplemental calories |

## END-STAGE RENAL FAILURE, CONTINUED

| Problem | Desired Outcome | Nursing Action/Order |
|---|---|---|
| Hiccups | D. No hiccups | 9. Medicate if ordered (Thorazine)<br>10. Give diversional activities<br>11. Symptomatic remedies, e.g. breathing $CO_2$ |
| GI bleeding | E. Stool, emesis, NG returns negative for blood | 12. Check stool, emesis, NG returns for evidence of blood (guaiac).<br>13. Increase frequency in observing vital signs.<br>14. Do not administer drugs containing aspirin. (Aspirin may cause GI ulceration and it prolongs clotting time) |
| X. Skin problems | A. Prevent scratching<br>B. Maintain the integrity of skin<br>C. Prevent further loss of moisture from skin | 1. Observe for pruitus, rashes, dryness or redness of skin, and for patient scratching<br>2. Use nondrying swabs, emollient/lanolin skin lotions<br>3. Bathe patient every other day, and use tepid water; pat skin dry<br>4. Keep patient's fingernails short<br>5. Provide cotton gloves or stockinette mittens, especially at night<br>6. Administer an antihistimine to decrease itching, if ordered<br>7. Use dry (powdered) shampoos to avoid drying with water; if hair is dry and brittle, oil treatments could be used<br>8. Use a humidifier during dry months |
| XI. Urinary problems | A. Accurate recordings of intake and output<br>B. Early detection of toxic side effects to medications<br>C. No urinary tract infections (UTI) | 1. Intake and output recording should include the time, amount and type of fluid<br>2. Assess patient for possible toxic side effects to drugs that could occur due to the renal failure and decreased urinary excretion (decreased hearing, decreased output)<br>3. Meticulous collection of urine cultures; monitor lab reports to assess presence of UTI.<br>4. Avoid use of urinary catheters; if used, prevent stasis of even minimal urine flow; position drainage tube to provide a patent, free-flowing system |

# END-STAGE RENAL FAILURE, CONTINUED

| Problem | Desired Outcome | Nursing Action/Order |
|---|---|---|
| XII. Musculoskeletal problems | A. No falls, fractures<br>B. Patient verbalizes that pain has decreased<br>C. Patient expresses a relief from muscle spasms<br>D. Patient demonstrates increasing tolerance of activity | 1. Provide safety precautions; assess needs for<br>a. Side rails<br>b. Assistance to ambulate<br>c. Assistive devices<br>d. Nonskid shoes/slippers<br>2. Develop a schedule for administration of the analgesic that meets each patient's needs<br>3. Assist patient to work out cramps by<br>Pushing against a food board<br>Standing<br>Pushing foot against nurse's hand<br>Using warm packs on legs<br>4. Assist with ambulation<br>5. Arrange for physical therapy follow-up to improve muscle tone |
| XIII. Endocrine problems<br>Altered sexual functioning | A. Patient understands that this is also related to renal function | 1. Establish a comfortable environment where the patient can discuss his or her feelings and problems |
| XIV. Hematopoietic problems<br>Diminished oxygen transport to the cells: fatigue, weakness, lethargy, dyspnea, chest pain | A. Establish the levels of activity the patient can tolerate<br>B. The patient can complete personal care without excessive fatigue, dyspnea or chest pain<br>C. No oral, GI or rectal bleeding; early detection if a problem occurs<br>D. Example: no more than 20 ml blood for lab tests every 24 hours.<br>E. Iron intake to help improve anemia | 1. Gradually increase level of activity to improve tolerance<br>2. Schedule cares activities with patient, include rest periods<br>3. Document when patient becomes excessively fatigued, dyspneic or has chest pain<br>4. Have patient avoid gas-forming foods<br>5. Elevate head of bed<br>6. $O_2$ whenever necessary for unrelieved dyspnea<br>7. Notify physician of unrelieved dyspnea or chest pain<br>8. Careful mouth care with a soft brush or gauze<br>9. Check stools for presence of blood<br>10. Administer stool softeners to avoid constipation<br>11. Schedule lab tests so an excessive amount of blood is not drawn at one time<br>12. Administer iron preparations if ordered; do not give them with a phosphate binder as this may interfere with its absorption |

## END-STAGE RENAL FAILURE, CONTINUED

| Problem | Desired Outcome | Nursing Action/Order |
|---|---|---|
| XV. Nutrition deficiency | A. Improve nutritional status by preventing GI losses and increasing diet intake | 1. Administer antiemetics 30–45 min before eating and whenever necessary<br>2. Schedule meal size and frequency with patient<br>3. Provide an environment conducive to eating |
| XVI. Infection | A. Prevention of any infection | 1. Aseptic care of all wounds, IV sites<br>2. Catheter care is provided, with perineal care minimum every 8 hours<br>3. Provide measures to prevent pneumonia: turn, cough, deep breathe, blow bottles, early ambulation<br>4. Assist the patient with oral and skin hygiene<br>5. Plan for ways to provide adequate nutrition<br>6. Obtain cultures as indicated |
| XVII. Psychologic problems<br>Fear of hospitalization and treatment procedures<br>Depression<br>Loss of strength and energy for self-care and life-role activities<br>Impairment of family relations and fullfilment of social needs | A. The patient's emotional and social needs are expressed and dealt with | 1. Work toward a nurse–patient relationship that is conducive to the patient expressing emotional and social needs<br>2. Insure the patient's right to privacy as well as free expression of needs<br>3. Self-care and independent functions are encouraged as soon as the patient can tolerate them<br>4. Keep the patient informed of his or her progress<br>5. Involve other disciplines in the patient's care and support: vocational rehabilitation counselor, financial counselor, chaplain, psychiatrist<br>6. Accept the patient's behavior as she or he tries to deal with the situation: anger, denial, mood swings |

## HEMODIALYSIS



| Problem | Desired Outcome | Nursing Action/Order |
|---|---|---|
| XVIII. Hemodialysis<br>Access care | A. Maintain patent access | 1. Check for patent flow every 4 hours:<br>Fistula—listen to and palpate the bruit<br>Shunt—check color, temperature of the tubing; listen for a bruit<br>2. Avoid activities and objects that compress the access extremity: blood pressure cuff, tight bandages, clothes, watchband, no venipunctures |
| | B. Prevent infection | 1. Aseptic, daily dressing changes of the external shunt with an antiseptic soap and sterile supplies; increase frequency of changes if the dressings get wet or if there is an infection<br>2. Observe for signs of infection: redness, tenderness, swelling, excessive warmth of skin |
| Hypotension during dialysis due to antihypertensive medication | C. No hypotension during dialysis due to rapid-acting drug | 1. Do not administer drugs that primarily or secondarily lower blood pressure without asking the physician |
| Hypotension postdialysis due to intravascular hypovolemia | D. Prevent shock and other injury during hypovolemia | 1. Help patient to slowly come to an upright position until the intracellular and intravascular volume reequilibrate: gradually elevate the head of the bed, get up slowly, call for assistance to get up |
| Potential bleeding due to heparinization | E. No bleeding | 1. No IM's until the effects of heparin wear off—4 hours<br>2. Check access sites for oozing; observe for blood in stool, emesis, incisions, wounds<br>3. Assist patient as needed to prevent bumps, cuts |
| Disequilibrium syndrome | F. Decrease fear of cerebral manifestations | 1. Especially in a new patient with a high BUN, observe for signs of: headache, nausea and vomiting, restlessness, confusion; check pulse, blood pressure and other neural signs<br>2. Provide a cool, quiet environment<br>3. Use seizure precautions<br>Medicate with analgesics or antiemetics |
| | G. Relieve nausea and vomiting, headache | 1. Medicate with analgesics or antiemetics |
| Hypokalemia | H. No complications due to decreased K+ | 1. Check for dysrhythmias, weakness<br>2. Give patient with a low postdialysis K+ a food high in K+, such as raisins, baked potato, banana |

## HEMODIALYSIS, CONTINUED

| Problem | Desired Outcome | Nursing Action/Order |
|---|---|---|
| Potential hepatitis | I. No hepatitis | 1. Isolate a patient with hepatitis from those without it<br>2. Use aseptic technique in handling all blood and excreta |
| Psychosocial changes<br>Dependent role<br>Family role reversal<br>Life-style changes | J. An environment is provided where the patient can work out feelings about these changes | 1. Work toward a nurse–patient relationship that is conducive to the patient expressing feelings<br>2. Self-care and independent functions are encouraged<br>3. Provide for time with appropriate resources such as a rehabilitation counselor<br>4. Accept the patient's behavior changes as he or she deals with changes |

## PERITONEAL DIALYSIS

| Problem | Desired Outcome | Nursing Action/Order |
|---|---|---|
| XIX. Peritoneal dialysis<br>Apprehension of procedure | A. Decreased apprehension | 1. Explain the procedure and its purpose<br>2. Sedate patient if ordered |
| Baseline vital signs | B. No omission of vital signs | 1. Check weight, blood pressure, pulse, temperature<br>2. Have patient void before catheter insertion |
| Catheter care | C. No infection | 1. Aseptic, daily dressing changes |
| Hypotension due to excess fluid removal | D. Avoid hypovolemia | 1. Carefully monitor blood pressure, pulse<br>2. Observe patient's behavior for restlessness, fear<br>3. Accurate recording of fluid balance is crucial in knowing the patient's status |
| Slow or no drainage | E. Rapid, free-flowing drainage phase | 1. Turn patient from side-to-side to reposition the catheter<br>2. Apply firm pressure to the abdomen<br>3. Elevate the head of the bed<br>4. Infuse a small amount of solution to dislodge possible fibrin blocking the catheter<br>5. Add heparin to the dialysate as ordered<br>6. Call physician to check catheter placement |
| Discomfort such as pain or chills | F. Decreased discomfort | 1. Warm dialysate to body temperature—37°C.<br>2. Assist patient to change position; give back-rubs<br>3. Administer analgesic<br>4. Provide diversional activity: TV, books |

## PERITONEAL DIALYSIS, CONTINUED

| Problem | Desired Outcome | Nursing Action/Order |
|---|---|---|
| Respiratory difficulty due to fluid, infection | G. No dyspnea, pain or infection | 1. Check rate and quality of respirations<br>2. Cough and hyperventilate frequently<br>3. Elevate head of bed to decrease pressure of dialysate on diaphragm<br>4. Stop infusion if acute distress<br>5. Provide small frequent feedings if food intake seems to increase dyspnea |
| Hyperglycemia | H. No hyperglycemia | 1. Monitor results of blood sugar levels<br>2. Adjust glucose level of dialysate as ordered |
| Peritonitis | I. No infection | 1. Rigid adherence to aseptic technique throughout the procedure: catheter insertion, warming and hanging of new bottles of solution, dressing changes<br>2. Culture dialysate fluid and catheter tip per physician order<br>3. Observe for signs of peritonitis: fever, tenderness or pain of abdomen |
| Protein loss | J. Minimize effects of loss | 1. Encourage diet intake of protein |

## TRANSPLANT

| Problem | Desired Outcome | Nursing Action/Order |
|---|---|---|
| XX. Transplantation<br>Fluid and electrolyte disturbance | A. Fluid intake is adjusted as the patient's output indicates | 1. Daily weight<br>2. Accurate I and O recordings: hourly to every 8 hours<br>3. IV to replace output ml for ml |
| | B. Imbalances detected early | 1. Vital signs every 2–4 hours (BP, P, CVP); monitor results of blood electrolytes<br>2. For continuing care, involve patient in doing own I and O, urine collection, BP, temperature |
| Infection due to immunosuppression<br>Wound, bladder, pneumonia | C. Protect patient from all sources of infection<br>No infection | 1. Aseptic care of wounds<br>2. Keep dressings dry<br>3. Special catheter and perineal care—minimum every 8 hours<br>4. Turn, cough, hyperventilate<br>5. Check changes in breath sounds<br>6. Assist with early ambulation<br>7. Special mouth care after all meals and h.s.<br>8. Restrict visitors: no one with colds or infections<br>9. Patient to wear gown and mask if leaving room |

## TRANSPLANT, CONTINUED

| Problem | Desired Outcome | Nursing Action/Order |
|---|---|---|
| Acute tubular necrosis (ATN) | D. Early detection of decreased renal function | 1. Assess for signs of ATN: increased weight, BP (fluid retention), BUN, creatinine, K+; decreased urinary output |
| Rejection | E. Early detection of rejection | 1. Assess for symptoms of rejection: low grade fever (100°F or higher), decreased urine output, increased blood pressure, tenderness over graft site |
| | F. Decrease of anxiety concerning loss of transplant and returning to dialysis | 2. Explain what rejection is and how it's treated<br>3. Allow time to ventilate feelings |
| Potential side effect due to high dose immunosupressive | G. Early detection of side effects<br>Provide emotional support | 1. Assess for<br>Depression, psychosis; ask patient about behavior changes<br>Hypertension<br>Leukopenia<br>Decreased wound healing<br>Increased bleeding time |
| Maintain integrity of patient's access | H. Access is available for use if dialysis is needed | 1. Continue to monitor for patency and infection<br>2. No BPs or drawing of blood or IV infusion |

This care plan was developed with the assistance of the nursing staff of B-6, Metropolitan Medical Center.

# APPENDIX C
# Patient Education Assessment

Date of interview: ______________________
Admission date: ______________________

Name: ______________________

Diagnosis: ______________________

Age: _____ Ethnic background: ______________________

Language other than English: ______________________

Family members who should be included:
______________________
______________________
______________________

**1. Readiness to learn**

Physical limitations:
- _______ Decreased vision
- _______ Decreased mental acuity
- _______ Fatigue
- _______ Anorexia
- _______ Decreased hearing
- _______ Sleeplessness

Stress level:
- _______ High (trembling, restless, pacing)
- _______ Low

Emotional limitations:
- _______ Lacks interest
- _______ Denial
- _______ Decreased initiative
- _______ Interested
- _______ Withdrawal
- _______ Has initiative

Cognitive:
- _______ Forgetful
- _______ Not oriented to planning for future
- _______ Preoccupied
- _______ Decreased concentration

**2. General intelligence**

Style of seeking information:
- _______ Active, asks questions
- _______ Passive, waits to be told
- _______ Both

Vocabulary:
- _______ Correct grammar
- _______ One syllable words
- Medical terminology—correct usage of medical terms: ____Yes ____No
- _______ Incorrect grammar
- _______ Multiple syllable words

Grade level attained. _______

Vocation/occupation: _______

Reading habits: _______ Books _______ Magazines _______ Newspapers

How do you spend your free time? ______________________

**3. Patient's understanding of illness and treatment**

Why are you hospitalized? ______________________

______________________

What do you think caused you to become sick? ______________________

______________________

What kind of symptoms have you had? ______________________________

______________________________

Have these symptoms restricted or changed your life?______________________________

______________________________

Are you currently on any restrictions? ______________________________

Diet: ______________________________

Activity: ______________________________

What medications are you taking? (Name, color, purpose—include over-the-counter):

______________________________

______________________________

______________________________

______________________________

______________________________

______________________________

______________________________

______________________________

**4. What the patient wants to learn**

_______More about the diagnosis    _______What it means for the future (prognosis)

Effect on: _____Family _____Work _____Social activities
_____Recreation _____Finances

More about: _____Treatment _____Diet _____Medications
_____Medical costs _____Other: ______________

Do you feel ready to begin learning about these things? ______________

**5. How the patient learns**

How do you like to learn new things?

__________ Reading    __________ Demonstrations    __________ With a group
__________ Pictures    __________ Doing it myself    __________ Alone
__________ TV
__________ Lectures
__________ Other: _______

**6. Teaching plan**

a. Readiness to learn:

b. Solutions to limitations:

c. Family to be included:

d. Who should teach:

e. Methods to use:

f. Topics and date for introduction to patient:

# APPENDIX D
# Renal Teaching Assessment

A. Medical management of end-stage renal disease (ESRD)

| | | Already knows | Needs review | Needs to learn |
|---|---|---|---|---|
| 1 | Self-care of daily weight | | | |
| 2 | Self-care of accurate I and O | | | |
| 3 | Collection of a 24-hour urine specimen | | | |
| 4 | Takes own blood pressure accurately | | | |
| 5 | Medications:<br>a. Name<br>b. Color<br>c. Purpose<br>d. How to take | | | |
| 6 | Diet restrictions:<br>a. Fluid<br>b. Protein<br>c. Sodium<br>d. Potassium<br>e. Other: | | | |
| 7 | Diagnosis | | | |

B. Dialysis-related topics (include A, 1–7)

| | | Already knows | Needs review | Needs to learn |
|---|---|---|---|---|
| 1 | Purpose of dialysis | | | |
| 2 | Access care:<br>a. Preop<br>b. Postop<br>c. Cannula dressing change<br>d. Fistula-maturing exercises<br>e. Peritoneal catheter care<br>f. Postdialysis | | | |
| 3 | Access complications:<br>a. Clotting<br>b. Infection<br>c. Hemorrhage | | | |
| 4 | Other | | | |

C. Transplantation-Related Topics (Include A, 1-7)

| | | Already knows | Needs review | Needs to learn |
|---|---|---|---|---|
| 1 | Work-up:<br>a. X rays<br>b. Crossmatch<br>c. Tissue type | | | |
| 2 | Surgery:<br>a. Nephrectomy<br>b. Splenectomy<br>c. Other: | | | |
| 3 | Transplant:<br>a. Site<br>b. Preop care<br>c. Postop care<br>d. Use of dialysis | | | |
| 4 | Immunosuppression:<br>a. Purpose<br>b. Schedule<br>c. Side effects | | | |
| 5 | Signs of rejection | | | |
| 6 | Signs of infection | | | |
| 7 | Activity posttransplant | | | |
| 8 | Self-care of temperature | | | |
| 9 | Self-care of wound — graft site | | | |
| 10 | Other | | | |